Carnivore Diet For Beginners + Cookbook

A Primal, Meat-Based Therapeutic Approach to Health and Wellness

George Kelly

Copyright © 2023 - All rights reserved

ISBN: 9798756412581

Legal Disclaimer

All the information presented in this book is for informational and educational purposes only.

It is not intended to provide medical advice or to take the place of such advice or treatment from a personal physician.

All readers/viewers of this content are advised to consult their doctors or qualified health professionals regarding specific health questions.

Neither George Kelly nor publisher of this content takes responsibility for possible health consequences of any person or persons reading or following the information in this educational content.

All viewers of this content, especially those taking prescription or over-the-counter medications, should consult their physicians before beginning any fitness, nutrition, supplement, or lifestyle program.

Contents

INTRODUCTION...8

CHAPTER 1: CARNIVORE DIET BASICS 101...........10

Carnivore Diet Foods......................................*10*

Carnivore Diet Spices......................................*12*

Carnivore Diet Snacks.....................................*16*

Do You Have To Eat Organ Meats?.....................*17*

Is Honey Carnivore?..*19*

Raw Milk On the Carnivore Diet.........................*23*

How Often Should You Eat On The Carnivore Diet?.....*26*

How Much Should You Eat On The Carnivore Diet?.....*27*

What Negative Symptoms You May Experience When First
Starting The Carnivore Diet?.........................*28*

How To Overcome Potentially Negative Symptoms When First
Starting The Carnivore Diet?.........................*28*

7-Day Carnivore Diet Meal Plan.........................*32*

Things to Consider Before Starting The Carnivore Diet.........*35*

How To Start The Carnivore Diet: Choose Your Level of Strictness..38

Mistakes To Avoid When First Starting The Carnivore Diet......41

Carnivore Diet Benefits...42

Carnivore Diet Drawbacks..47

CHAPTER 2: KETO VS CARNIVORE DIET...........................**50**

What Is The Keto Diet?...50

What Is The Carnivore Diet?..51

Differences Between Keto and Carnivore..................................53

Similarities Between Keto and Carnivore..................................56

Alternating Between Keto and Carnivore..................................58

How To Transition From Keto To Carnivore............................59

Keto vs Carnivore: Which Diet Is Better?.................................61

CHAPTER 3: VEGAN VS CARNIVORE DIET...........................**62**

What Is The Vegan Diet?...63

Is The Vegan Diet Healthy?...63

Vegan Nutrient Deficiencies..65

What Do the Vegan and Carnivore Diets Have in Common?......89

CHAPTER 4: CARNIVORE DIET AND AUTOIMMUNITY..........**90**

Why Does The Carnivore Diet Work So Well For Autoimmunity?..................90

CHAPTER 5: CARNIVORE DIET RECIPES...........................**98**

Snacks & Appetizers...........................98

Main Dishes...........................119

Desserts...........................137

CHAPTER 6: CARNIVORE DIET FAQS...........................**141**

Why Does The Carnivore Diet Work So Well?...........................141

Who Should Follow The Carnivore Diet?...........................142

What Are The Potential Benefits Of The Carnivore Diet For Autoimmune Patients?...........................142

Can The Carnivore Diet Heal Autoimmune Disease?...........................143

Is The Carnivore Diet Safe Long-Term?...........................143

What Are The People's Results From Using The Carnivore Diet?...........................144

What's The Easiest Way to Start The Carnivore Diet?...........................145

Is Meat Healthy?...........................145

Do We Really Need Vegetables To Stay Healthy?...........................147

What About Fiber On The Carnivore Diet?...........................147

Is The Carnivore Diet Ketogenic?...........................148

Can The Carnivore Diet Cause Nutrient Deficiencies? If Yes, How To Prevent Them?.................149

Does The Carnivore Diet Increase Serum Cholesterol?.............152

Can The Carnivore Diet Cause Constipation?..................152

What Are The Most Common Digestive Problems When First Starting The Carnivore Diet?.................153

Can Eating Too Much Meat Cause Kidney Problems?.................153

How Long Does It Take To Adapt To The Carnivore Diet?.......154

Can I Use Supplements When Following The Carnivore Diet?.................154

Does The Carnivore Diet Work For Athletes?..................155

Can You Build Muscle While On The Carnivore Diet?.................155

Is Weight Loss Easier On The Carnivore Diet?.................155

Is it a Good Idea to Eat Meat as a Pre-Workout Meal?.............156

Can You Eat Carbs While On The Carnivore Diet?.................156

What Is The Best Diet For Healing Autoimmunity?..................157

CONCLUSION.................**159**

REFERENCES.................**162**

INTRODUCTION

One of the most controversial topics of debate among scientists and the general population alike is what is the ideal diet for optimum human health, longevity and performance. It's estimated that nearly 50% of the American adult population attempts to lose weight at some point every year. Most people recognize that one of the primary ways to lose weight is by changing your diet.

Yet, the sheer number of diet plans available to us makes it very difficult to even start, as there is great uncertainty about which one is better suited for us, more effective, and sustainable long-term. Every diet seems to have a different objective: some diets aim to curb our appetite to reduce our food intake, while others suggest restricting our intake of calories and either carbs or fat. What's more, many diets seem to offer health benefits that go beyond just weight loss.

One such example of a diet with various purported health benefits and applications - from weight loss, improved gut health, optimized body composition, enhanced mental and cognitive performance, autoimmune healing, etc, that has gained extreme popularity in the recent years is the carnivore diet.

The carnivore diet, as the name implies, is an exclusively animal-based diet that consists almost entirely of meat, such as red meat, fish and poultry. Eggs and dairy products are also sometimes permitted depending on the carnivore diet variation.

The carnivore diet excludes completely all plant foods, including fruits, vegetables, nuts, seeds, grains, and legumes, as well as all plant by-products, such as olive oil, coconut oil, avocado oil, nut butters, etc.

CHAPTER 1: CARNIVORE DIET BASICS 101

The carnivore diet is a high-fat, high-protein diet where you are allowed to eat only animal foods and eliminate all plant-based foods. By cutting out all plant foods, you essentially remove almost all carbohydrates, so your body will now have to rely solely on protein and fats for its energy and calories.

Carnivore Diet Foods

The carnivore diet includes the following foods:
• **Meat:** Beef, Veal, Lamb, Sheep, Buffalo, Venison, Deer, Antelope, Kangaroo, Pork, Chicken, Turkey, Duck, Goose, Ostrich, Wild Game.
• **Fish:** Salmon, Cod, Sardines, Herring, Halibut, Atlantic Mackerel, Tuna, Lake Trout, Bass, Freshwater Whitefish, Tilapia, Sole, Anchovy, Arctic Char.
• **Seafood:** Shrimp, Octopus, Abalone, Eel, Clam, Crab, Crayfish, Lobster, Oyster, Scallop, Squid, Cuttlefish, Fish Roe.
• **Other Animal Foods:** Eggs, Bone Marrow.
• **Animal Fat:** Tallow, Lard, Duck Fat, Suet.
• **Dairy:** Butter, Ghee, Cream, Raw Milk, Cheese, Yogurt, Kefir.
• **Sugars:** Raw Honey (some carnivore diet variations exclude honey altogether)
• **Salt:** Sea Salt, Himalayan Pink Salt.

• **Beverages:** Water, Bone broth.

The carnivore diet prohibits the following foods:
• **Fruits:** Apples, Bananas, Oranges, Berries, Pears, Peaches, Plums.
• **Veggies:** Broccoli, Cauliflower, Spinach, Kale, Zucchini, Tomatoes, Bell Peppers.
• **Legumes:** Chickpeas, Kidney Beans, Black Beans, Lentils, Pinto Beans.
• **Nuts:** Almonds, Walnuts, Macadamia Nuts, Pecans, Cashews, Pistachios.
• **Seeds:** Chia Seeds, Flax Seeds, Pumpkin Seeds, Hemp Seeds, Sunflower Seeds.
• **Grains:** Amaranth, Quinoa, Wheat, Buckwheat, Rice, Oats, Barley, Pasta.
• **Processed foods:** Chips, Crackers, Cookies, Candy, Convenience Meals, Fast Food.
• **Beverages:** Tea, Coffee, Cocoa, Sports Drinks, Sodas, Energy Drinks.
• **Sugars:** Table Sugar, Brown Sugar, Maple Syrup.

Despite all the food limitations that the carnivore diet imposes, one of its most alluring aspects is that you don't have to track anything - no food logging, counting macros, calculating calories, or timing meals. As long as the food you eat comes from an animal source, you can eat it whenever you want, and as much as you want! Or, as many carnivore proponents like to put it, all you have to do is "Eat meat. Drink water."
In general, when following the carnivore diet, you'll want to emphasize the fattier cuts of meat and less so the lean cuts. This will help you get the right amount of calories and nutrients, as

well as maintain optimal hormonal balance and body composition. The saturated fats and cholesterol found abundantly in animal foods are precursor substances to steroid hormones, such as corticosteroids and sex steroids (androgens, estrogens, and progestogens).

Carnivore Diet Spices

A 100% strict carnivore diet usually does not involve any herbs or spices. For this diet, salt is used for electrolytes and suffices for seasoning. Surprisingly, most people are satisfied with this and achieve great health and body composition results by using high-quality salt alone.

The decision to use or not use spices will depend on the individual's context, goals, gut health status, and intolerance to specific foods. The use of spices also comes down to the individual's sensitivities to compounds such as oxalates and lectins present in them. Herbs and spices fall on a spectrum with some being highly inflammatory and others less inflammatory. The carnivore diet is by default very effective at lowering inflammation and you don't want to counteract that by including the wrong types of spices. One of the reasons people find such great success on the carnivore diet is because they eliminate all inflammatory plant foods.

In a diet that is based around meat and animal foods, herbs and spices should be consumed only in trace amounts, if at all. Even trace amounts of the wrong spice can trigger negative reactions. The problems that arise from consuming certain herbs and spices are due to anti-nutrients. Anti-nutrients are plant defense compounds that bind to minerals, irritate the gut, stimulate the immune system and cause negative symptoms in the body, such as mineral deficiencies, kidney stones, leaky gut, and exacerbate pre-existing autoimmune conditions.

When it comes to using herbs and spices on the carnivore diet, the ones recommended are those that are low in anti-nutrients, such as oxalates and lectins.

Oxalates: People who are sensitive to oxalates experience symptoms, such as kidney stones, fibromyalgia (systemic pain and increased sensitivity to pain) and thyroid dysfunction. If you have any of these conditions or you know you are sensitive to oxalates, here are the spices you should probably avoid and some other ones that may be okay for you.

High-Oxalate Herbs & Spices
• Cinnamon
• Turmeric
• Black Pepper
• Cumin Seed
• Fennel Seed
• Allspice

Low-Oxalate Herbs & Spices
• Garlic Powder
• White Pepper
• Basil
• Cilantro
• Vanilla
• Mustard
• Thyme
• Red Pepper Flakes
• Paprika

- Cardamon
- Chilli Powder
- Cayenne Pepper

Lectins: People sensitive to lectins may experience the following symptoms when consuming foods that contain them: bloating, gas, indigestion, digestive disturbances, IBS, leaky gut and other autoimmune symptoms, such as rheumatoid arthritis (RA). A family of plants that notoriously contain high levels of lectins are nightshades. Nightshades include:

- **Fruits:** Tomatoes, Tomatillos, Pimentos, Bell Peppers, Jalapeno Peppers, Habanero Peppers, Chili Peppers, Cape Gooseberry, Naranjilla, Garden Huckleberry.
- **Vegetables:** Potatoes, Eggplants.
- **Berries:** Goji Berries, Gooseberries, Ashwagandha.
- **Spices and Sauces:** Cayenne, Chili, Curry, Paprika, Cumin, Mustard, Tomato Sauce, Marinara Sauce, Ketchup.

If you are sensitive to lectins you should avoid herbs and spices that contain high levels of them.

High-Lectin Herbs and Spices
- Paprika
- Chili Pepper Flakes
- Cayenne Pepper
- Cumin
- Peppermint
- Nutmeg
- Chilli Powder
- Curry Powder

Low-Lectin Herbs and Spices
• Onion Powder
• Chives
• Fennel
• Parsley
• Basil
• Mint
• Cilantro
• Rosemary
• Sage
• Tarragon
• Thyme
• Oregano
• Ginger
• Sage

Best Carnivore Herbs & Spices
• Basil
• Bay Leaf
• Parsley
• Sage
• Vanilla Bean
• Rosemary
• Thyme
• Dill
• Cilantro
• Chines
• Tarragon
• Oregano
• Ginger
• Garlic

Worst Carnivore Herbs & Spices

- Red Chili Flakes
- Chilli Powder
- Curry Powder
- Cumin Seed
- Dill Seed
- Fennel Seed
- Cardamom
- Coriander Seed
- Nutmeg
- Mustard Seed

In general, the least inflammatory herbs and spices are going to be leaves and the most inflammatory are going to be seeds. When you buy any herb or spice, make sure it's organic, it doesn't contain added fillers, and is fresh.

Carnivore Diet Snacks

For optimal metabolic health and body composition, it's generally recommended to fast long and eat only big, solid meals, eliminating the habit of snacking altogether. This is particularly applicable if your main goals include fat loss, autoimmune recovery, or optimizing longevity. Saying that, at some point, you may find yourself hungry but not able to have a complete, full meal. In such cases, you should grab a carnivore-approved snack to tide you over and raise your blood sugar a bit until the time of your normal meal comes. Many of the following carnivore-approved snacks are also shelf-stable and good to stock up on as healthy, low-carb emergency foods.

Carnivore-Approved Snacks
• Pemmican
• Liver chips
• Bone broth
• Pickled eggs
• Mini meat pies
• Beef jerky and meat sticks
• Liverwurst
• Canned fish
• Pork rinds

Do You Have To Eat Organ Meats?

Good question! Organs are by far the most nutrient-dense parts of the animal, however, some people can't seem to be able to tolerate their taste. These people usually like to stick to muscle meat only when following the carnivore diet, while others choose to include organ meats and discover recipes to cook them in ways that are tasty and palatable.

Animal organs and other parts of the animal, such as bones and fat often provide nutrients that fuel the same organs or parts in our own body. This principle of "like heals like" is the basis of glandular therapy. Glandular therapy uses whole animal tissues (organs primarily) to heal or enhance the functioning of the body's corresponding tissues.

All organs and glands of an animal contain enzymes, vitamins, minerals, trace elements, peptides, nucleotides, and other bioactive factors specific to that organ or gland. The consumption of the corresponding organ or gland from a healthy animal promotes the healthy functioning of that particular organ/gland in our body (homostimulation). That's because vitamins and minerals are found primarily in tissues where they are used the most.

For example, B vitamins that support detoxification and energy production are found in the liver – the body's main detoxification organ. Calcium and phosphorus are found in the bones and teeth of animals, and support human bone and teeth health when consumed in the form of bone broth. Pancreatic enzymes are found abundantly in the pancreas of animals and support human digestion and pancreatic health when ingested raw (as in freeze-dried capsules), because all enzymes are heat-sensitive

In opposition to today's eating practices, eating nose-to-tail was actually the norm for our ancestors who didn't have a butcher to go to and order a ribeye whenever they wanted. Our ancestors recognized the immense nutritional and energetic value of organ meats (offal). Even in pre-history, early hominids depended on the energy, nutrients and fatty acids contained in organ meats. In the table below, you can see the calories, fat, protein and fatty acid profile of various foods available to early hominids.

As you can see, no one food contains sufficient amounts of all three: fatty acids, calories and protein. The highest energy foods, like marrow, are devoid of DHA. The highest protein foods are devoid of fat and DHA. And the highest foods in DHA do not offer sufficient energy (calories). The only way to get all of them in sufficient quantities was by consuming the entire animal, nose-to-tail.

Table 2. Comparison of energy density, protein content and arachidonic acid (AA) and docosahexaenoic acid (DHA) in food sources (100 g samples) available to early hominids

Food	Energy kcal	Fat g	Protein g	AA mg	DHA mg	DHA/ energy mg/kcal	DHA/ protein mg/g
African ruminant brain[a]	126	9.3	9.8	533	861	6.83	87.86
African freshwater fish[b]	119	4.5	18.8	270	549	4.61	29.20
African ruminant liver[c]	159	7.1	22.6	192	41	0.27	1.81
African ruminant muscle[d]	113	2.1	22.7	152	10	0.09	0.45
Ruminant marrow[e]	488	51.0	7.0	n.d.[i]	n.d.	–	–
African ruminant subcutaneous fat[f]	745	82.3	1	20–180	trace[j]	–	–
Wild tubers/roots[g]	96	0.5	2.0	n.d.	n.d.	–	–
Wild nuts[g]	306	29.0	13.0	n.d.	n.d.	–	–
Mixed, edible wild plant foods[h]	129	2.8	4.1	n.d.	n.d.	–	–

[a] Derived from [13, 29, 30], [b] derived from [28], [c] derived from [27], [d] derived from [27], [e] derived from [29–31], [f] derived from [26], [g] derived from [37, 38], [h] derived from [35], [i] n.d. (not detectable), [j] trace (less than 0.01% of total fatty acids).

Is Honey Carnivore?

Honey is very rich in carbohydrates, specifically glucose, fructose and sucrose. There's nothing inherently wrong with carbohydrates, but some people shouldn't include them in their diet when trying to heal their body and gut. As an example, if you suffer from SIBO or yeast overgrowth, you should abstain from honey completely for some time. Most of the time, the inclusion of honey in the carnivore diet is a hot and debated topic.

Honey is an animal-based product derived from insects within the animal kingdom, but the product itself, honey, doesn't contain any animal tissue or cells like dairy products, which are carnivore-friendly foods coming from animals. Thus, if you follow a strict, zero-carb carnivore diet, honey shouldn't be part of your diet. On the opposite, if you are an athlete, honey may comprise a great, gut-friendly, easy-to-digest, and nutritious source of fuel and micronutrients for you. One of the main benefits of the carnivore diet is the elimination principle. A lot of people have food-related diseases or challenges, and by just eliminating plants they see great relief. Thus, if you are a complete newbie to the carnivore diet, it is recommended you exclude honey altogether at the start and strategically introduce it at some point later.

How Honey Is Made?

Honey starts as flower nectar collected by bees, which gets broken down into simple sugars stored inside the honeycomb. The design of the honeycomb and constant fanning of the bees' wings causes evaporation, creating sweet liquid honey. Honey's color and flavor may vary based on the type of nectar collected by the bees. For example, honey made from orange blossom nectar might be light in color, whereas honey from avocado or wildflowers might have a dark amber color.

On average, a hive will produce about 65 pounds of surplus honey each year. Beekeepers harvest it by collecting the honeycomb frames and scraping off the wax cap that bees make to seal off honey in each cell. Once the caps are removed, the frames are placed in an extractor, which is a centrifuge that spins the frames, forcing honey out of the comb.

After the honey is extracted, it's strained to remove any remaining wax and other particles. Some beekeepers and bottlers might heat the honey to make this process easier, even though raw (unheated) honey is always superior from a nutrition and health standpoint.

Is Honey Healthier Than Sugar?

Honey is a naturally-derived sweetener and thus, a healthier alternative to processed sugar. One of the reasons for that is that table sugar is a processed food product where all the nutrients, vitamins, minerals and enzymes have been removed. When you eat sugar your body is forced to compensate for the missing nutrients by mobilizing its own nutrient reserves. That promotes nutritional deficiencies and increased levels of inflammation.

For example, some people may develop magnesium and potassium deficiencies as a result of eating too much sugar because these minerals are necessary for carb metabolism. Magnesium and potassium deficiencies can seriously undermine your health: they can spike your blood pressure and blood sugar, as well as cause neurological and behavioral malfunctions. Honey, on the other hand, contains small amounts of magnesium and other micronutrients, which make it a healthier, more nutritious dietary addition to processed sugar.

Some Of The Healthiest People In The World Consume Large Amounts Of Honey

Honey is the most energy-dense food found in nature. Thus, it is not surprising that where it exists honey is an important food for almost all hunter-gatherers. For example, raw honey and bee products in general have a very special role in the Hadza tribe diet. This African tribe of hunter-gatherers residing in central Tanzania is the most extensively studied nomadic group in the world. In the last couple of years, the Hadza tribe diet has gained extreme popularity among health circles around the world due to its purported gut health and longevity-promoting benefits.

The Hadza group resides in a tropical forest and their diet consists of plants, fruits, tubers, and game animals. During the dry season, the Hadza people eat much more meat, while in the wet season much more berries and especially honey. More specifically, the Hadza women acquire honey that is close to the ground, while men climb tall baobab trees to raid the largest bee hives with stinging bees. Overall, honey accounts for a substantial proportion of the kilocalories (kcal) in the Hadza diet, especially that of Hadza men.

Benefits of Raw Honey

Raw honey has been used as a folk remedy throughout history as it offers a variety of well-established health benefits and medical applications. Today, honey is even used in some hospitals as a treatment for wounds. Many of the health benefits of honey are specific to raw or unpasteurized honey.

Most of the honey we find in the grocery store is pasteurized. The high heat kills unwanted bacteria and yeast, may improve the color and texture, removes any crystallization, and extends honey's shelf life. At the same time, many of the beneficial nutrients and enzymes are destroyed.

Raw honey, especially raw dark honey, is also a great source of antioxidants. It contains an array of plant phytochemicals that act as free radical scavengers (antioxidants). Some types of raw honey have as many antioxidants as fruits and vegetables, which is fascinating. Antioxidants help protect our body from cell damage caused by free radicals, such as reactive oxygen species (ROS).

Free radicals contribute to the aging and inflammatory process in our body, and may promote the development of various chronic diseases, including cancer, neurodegenerative disorders, and heart disease. Research shows that antioxidant compounds present in raw honey called polyphenols exert a protective effect against heart disease and other chronic inflammatory diseases. Raw honey also carries antibacterial and antifungal properties. Research has shown that raw honey can kill unwanted bacteria and fungi as it naturally contains hydrogen peroxide (H_2O_2), an antiseptic. Its effectiveness as an antibacterial or antifungal agent varies depending on the honey, but it's clearly more than a folk remedy for these kinds of infections. Concerning its macronutrient profile, a tablespoon of honey has about 64 total calories, 17 g of net carbohydrates, 0.1 g of protein, but 0 g of fat or fiber.

Some of the vitamins found in honey include ascorbic acid (vitamin C), pantothenic acid (vitamin B5), niacin (vitamin B3) and riboflavin (vitamin B2), along with minerals such as calcium, copper, iron, magnesium, manganese, phosphorus, potassium and zinc.

Raw Milk On the Carnivore Diet

Milk is a nutrient-rich liquid food produced by the mammary glands of mammals. It is the primary source of nutrition for young mammals. For those following the carnivore diet, raw milk is an excellent source of animal-based carbs, primarily lactose. Due to its high calorie and nutrient content, raw milk is very beneficial for building muscle and gaining weight. It is also very useful for correcting nutrient deficiencies, especially for those recovering from long-term restrictive diets or anorexics. Raw milk is specified over pasteurized milk due to the enzymes, probiotics and heat-sensitive enzymes it contains, that get otherwise destroyed during pasteurization.

Raw Milk Benefits

People have been drinking raw milk straight from their cows, sheep, and goats for millennia. Raw milk has long been one of the most nutritionally complete foods in the human diet and an integral component of nearly every culture's cuisine. In today's super-sanitized, germophobic and technologically advanced world, raw milk is irrationally demonized for various reasons.

Dairy, especially cow dairy, can indeed be problematic for a lot of people. However, dairy derived from goats, sheep, or buffalo is much more gut and immune-friendly due to the chemical structure of casein (milk protein) it contains. On top of that, many individuals who normally are lactose intolerant often find that they can tolerate raw milk just fine. These people actually have a pasteurization intolerance, not a dairy intolerance.

A reason that this happens is that raw milk naturally contains the enzyme lactase and specific probiotic species, like *Lactococcus, Lactobacillus, Leuconostoc, Streptococcus* and *Enterococcus* which break down lactose, a disaccharide found in milk, into galactose and glucose, which are digestible, simple sugars. Raw milk has for decades been well-regarded in health circles due to its unique health-promoting benefits:

• Raw milk provides readily available nutritional elements our body needs for repair and regeneration, including easily assimilable proteins and fats in their whole, unprocessed, unadulterated form.

• The fatty acids in raw milk nourish the brain and intestinal lining, and upregulate mitochondrial function. Mitochondria are membrane-bound cell organelles that generate most of the chemical energy needed to power the cell's biochemical reactions.

• Raw milk contains the enzyme phosphatase and other crucial enzymes necessary for the complete absorption of calcium, which are not present in pasteurized milk. That's why some research papers (falsely) link dairy consumption with the onset, rather than the prevention, of osteoporosis.

• Naturally-occurring beneficial bacteria (probiotics) in raw milk carry amazing benefits for our gut, immune and digestive health.

• Raw milk is a perfect source of unheated, unoxidized cholesterol, fatty acids, and non-denatured proteins. Protein denaturing or protein denaturation is a change in the chemical structure of protein that occurs due to chemical effects. The most common source of protein denaturing is heat application, as happens in pasteurization and cooking.

• Raw milk is nature's perfect electrolyte drink. It contains large amounts of organic minerals, which nourish the body's organs, glands and tissues, provide intracellular hydration and optimize brain function.

• Colostrum (first mammal's milk after birth), but raw milk as well, contain immunoglobulins/antibodies, and complement factors that upregulate immune function and provide major antimicrobial effects against a wide range of pathogens.

• People with bone-related conditions, like bone spurs, osteopenia and osteoporosis, notice their condition significantly improving or completely disappearing after a few months of daily ingestion of fresh, raw milk.

Where to Find Raw Milk?
Raw milk is not the easiest product to obtain, since its distribution in many countries and U.S states is illegal. Many food and drug administrations around the world state that raw

milk is particularly fertile for germs because it is unpasteurized, therefore not safe for human consumption.

This may apply to poor quality raw milk coming from unsanitary, industrially-raised animals. Raw milk sourced from healthy and happy ruminants naturally contains anti-microbial enzymes and probiotics that antagonize and inhibit pathogenic bacteria proliferation, such as *Salmonella, E. coli, Listeria, Campylobacter* and others that cause foodborne illness, also known as "food poisoning."

A good way to access raw milk (if the legal route is not an option), is by asking local farmers whether they might sell you some directly. Realmilk.com is a great resource for learning about the safety and health benefits of raw milk. Realmilk.com also includes a searchable database of farmers that sell raw milk around the world.

How Often Should You Eat On The Carnivore Diet?

There is no right or wrong way to approach your eating frequency while on the carnivore diet. Eating as often and as much as you need to feel full and satiated is a good rule to follow. If you prefer to spread your meals over the day, you may stick to three solid meals per day or two meals and a snack.

On the other hand, if you like to incorporate some intermittent fasting into your daily routine, you may do two or even one meal a day (OMAD). If you are an athlete with increased caloric/nutritional needs, you may find that two or three meals during the day help you spread out your protein intake better than OMAD, in order to optimally support your athletic endeavors.

How Much Should You Eat On The Carnivore Diet?

The most common answer is to eat as much as you like until you feel full. Meat is incredibly filling and you'll be surprised how easy it will be going for many hours without eating. Meat digests much slower than most foods, especially carbs, meaning it will be a lot easier for you to control your cravings and food intake during the day. Thus, the carnivore diet apart from decreasing inflammation and correcting nutrient deficiencies, it may also help you achieve your fat loss goals faster.

The average carnivore diet meal plan typically consists of two pounds of meat per day, coming primarily from ruminant, polygastric animals, such as beef, lamb, goat, sheep, buffalo, etc. You will likely want (and should) eat much more meat during the first month on the diet, as your digestive system and appetite slowly adjust, and you start fighting your cravings for other foods.

Once you have adjusted to the diet a bit, you may start tracking your calories and levels of physical activity depending on your body composition goals: do you want to build muscle or lose some fat? If you hit the gym every day and want to bulk up, then four or more pounds of meat per day is not uncommon, and oftentimes necessary.

What Negative Symptoms You May Experience When First Starting The Carnivore Diet?

Common negative side effects you may experience when starting the carnivore diet include:
• Brain fog or trouble focusing
• Headaches
• Dehydration
• Mood swings
• Disrupted bowel movements (constipation or diarrhea)
• Nausea
• Indigestion
• Fatigue
• Insomnia
• Dehydration
• Food cravings

How To Overcome Potentially Negative Symptoms When First Starting The Carnivore Diet?

Since you now know what negative side effects you may expect when first starting the carnivore diet, it's time to learn some tips and tricks to overcome them:

1. Eat More Meat
Feeling hungry during the first couple of weeks on the carnivore diet is not uncommon. The last thing you should do is ignore those hunger signals. If you find that you feel hungry in

the beginning, you can do one of those two things (or both): eat more meat or eat better quality meat. If you buy organic, pasture-raised, grass-fed beef as opposed to conventional, feedlot beef, you'll get more nutrients and less toxins from the same amount of food volume. This will result in more energy, less cravings, better mood, accelerated muscle recovery, and improved levels of well-being. When it comes to sourcing your meats, you may consider the following meat delivery services:
• Crowd Cow
• Butcher Box
• Honest Bison

2. Don't Neglect Water

As already mentioned, in the first couple of days you will experience a significant amount of water loss due to your glycogen reserves being depleted and used as energy. This is a normal physiologic process that occurs when your diet lacks carbs and fiber which normally attract water. This process alone can remove four to six pounds of water from your body that needs to be replenished somehow.

Along with the water, you'll also lose lots of electrolytes, especially sodium, potassium and magnesium, which may induce further dehydration and cause negative symptoms, such as headaches, fatigue, brain fog, and muscle cramps. To counteract those side effects, aim at a minimum of one pint of filtered water three times a day, along with 2 extra pints in between.

3. Use Electrolytes

You can keep track of all the nutrition you get in terms of calories, protein, carbs, fats, etc, but evaluating your electrolyte intake can be a little more challenging. Salt generally has a terrible name, and most people believe you should keep it to a minimum when on a restrictive diet. That, however, could not be further from the truth.

When you follow an omnivore diet that is diverse and includes many different types of vegetables rich in minerals/electrolytes, such as leafy greens, cruciferous vegetables, squashes, etc, you can get away with reducing your salt intake much easier. That doesn't apply when you eat a strict meat-only carnivore diet that is naturally low in potassium and magnesium. So, to prevent any electrolyte deficiencies and/or dehydration, you should salt your food liberally and use an electrolyte powder rich in potassium in order to cover your mineral needs. Take a few servings, and you'll be all set with less guesswork involved.

4. Support Your Digestion & Elimination

Digestive problems that can occur when first starting following the carnivore diet can oftentimes be very disruptive, even more so than suffering for a couple of days from brain fog and low energy. Some people may experience bloating and indigestion, while others constipation or diarrhea. The far more common problem is diarrhea.

This is because the gallbladder is not able to produce enough bile to deal with the increased intake of dietary fats. As a result, some of the fat passes undigested through the digestive tract causing diarrhea. To solve this issue, one option is to reduce your dietary fat intake. The other option is to supplement with digestive aids like ox bile, pancreatic lipase **or** betaine HCL to help your body process and break down dietary fat.

5. Get Enough Sleep

This is one aspect a lot of people don't focus enough on. As you adjust how you eat, especially in a carnivorous way, you can easily end up focusing way too much on nutrition and not so much on lifestyle and other aspects of health. Oftentimes, the solution to many of the problems that occur on the carnivore diet, including some of the aforementioned side effects, is simply getting enough quality sleep. Even an extra hour or two in bed can make a huge difference in how you feel and perform.

Tips to Improve Sleep:

1. Sleep in a pitch-dark, cool room and open a window for ventilation purposes.

2. Turn off the lights by 11 pm

3. Don't exercise close to bedtime, as this will increase the production of stress hormones, such as cortisol and adrenaline, and elevate your blood pressure, which will prevent your body from toning down and relaxing.

4. No screen time after 10 pm, but reading a book is fine and actually beneficial for helping you fall asleep faster.

5. No liquids after 9 pm to avoid getting up in the middle of the night to pee (nocturia).

These tips will help set up the right conditions for a good night's sleep and assist you in waking up fully refreshed and ready to dig into that morning steak.

6. Stay Active And Sweat More

Being more active while on the carnivore diet will not only help you with your weight loss goals, but in other aspects of health as well. That's because several processes in the body are triggered by physical activity. Moving your body enough will result in better blood flow and oxygen delivery to all tissues of your body, as well as faster and more efficient digestion.

On top of that, physical exercise will help increase your appetite, making you want to eat more. And more meat will mean more nutrients, improved athletic performance and better cognition. Finally, you will sweat a lot more, and sweating is an excellent way for your body to expel toxins that may have built up through years of poor eating habits. Moreover, removing toxins will reduce the inflammatory burden of your body and reduce your risk of all sorts of chronic diseases.

7-Day Carnivore Diet Meal Plan

It's impossible to follow a diet like carnivore without a little bit of pre-planning and preparation. Thus, you'll want to come up with a meal plan and figure out what sort of foods you'll be eating for every meal of the day. Once you've put together a meal plan, you can assemble a grocery list and purchase the foods you'll need during the week. Most people that follow this diet do some sort of meal prep so that they have the time to eat fresh food every day. For example, many people cook up meals in advance, freeze them, and then warm them when they're ready to eat. If you look at this sample menu below, you will get an idea in order to be able to put together a meal plan that will work best for you.

BREAKFAST

Breakfast is oftentimes considered the most important meal of the day. This is true when it's the only meal of the day. While some people avoid breakfast altogether, there are plenty of carnivore-friendly options for your first meal of the day. A good example would be:

- **Day 1:** Steak and eggs
- **Day 2:** Feta cheese omelette
- **Day 3:** Poached eggs with bacon
- **Day 4:** Kefir and two eggs over medium
- **Day 5:** Chicken livers and scrambled eggs
- **Day 6:** Chicken and feta omelette
- **Day 7:** Bacon and eggs

LUNCH

A lot of people eat lunch at work, which means that they grab fast food or takeout. This isn't an option when following the carnivore diet, which is why you'll want to plan ahead and bring carnivore-friendly, animal-based foods with you:

- **Day 1:** Salmon and fried pork
- **Day 2:** Chicken thighs with cheddar cheese
- **Day 3:** Tuna and hard-boiled eggs
- **Day 4:** Shredded chicken with bacon
- **Day 5:** Turkey burgers
- **Day 6:** Beef liver
- **Day 7:** Grilled chicken tenders

SNACKS

Since many of the meals on the carnivore diet don't include side dishes, you may need to supplement your diet with some sort of snacks. Thankfully, there are more options for snacks on this diet than most people realize:

- **Day 1:** Cottage cheese
- **Day 2:** Liver chips
- **Day 3:** Sardines
- **Day 4:** Tuna
- **Day 5:** Hard-boiled eggs
- **Day 6:** Sardines
- **Day 7:** Steak bites

DINNER

It's important to finish off your day with a nice, filling meal that will leave you happy, satiated, and energized until the next morning. A good general tip to follow is to eat your last meal of the day several hours before bedtime. That's because eating later during the day disrupts sleep and hinders digestion. There are plenty of excellent dinnertime options for people following the carnivore diet:

- **Day 1:** Ground beef patties
- **Day 2:** Ribeye steak
- **Day 3:** Bone broth and roasted chicken
- **Day 4:** Bison burgers
- **Day 5:** Slow-roasted salmon
- **Day 6:** Pork chops
- **Day 7:** Prime rib

Because meat and seafood can be expensive, it's important to plan ahead and develop a meal plan that will allow you to reuse the same types of meat in different ways. For example, you could have bacon and eggs for breakfast, eat bacon-wrapped chicken for lunch, and have roasted chicken at dinnertime.

It's also frequently recommended that people who are new to the carnivore diet should focus on steak and other types of red meat over poultry, as these types of meat contain more fat, calories and nutrients, and are lower in the pro-inflammatory omega-6 fatty acids. Once your body has adjusted to the diet, you may experiment more with your meal plan and include a greater variety of meats and animal products.

Things to Consider Before Starting The Carnivore Diet

There are a few things you need to consider before jumping into this radically new lifestyle and way of eating. While the instructions you have to follow are quite simple, their application is not always easy.

1. Living Without Eating Any Plants

A meat-only diet is a lifestyle choice that is easier said than done. Even for the biggest meat and BBQ lover out there, completely avoiding plant foods altogether is a lot more difficult and complicated than it sounds.

If you've ever kept a food journal, you will have regularly added snacks like apples or bananas, or even some granola or nut protein bars. Well, these will be all gone when following a strict carnivore diet. The same applies to this delicious cookie you oftentimes enjoy with your afternoon coffee. The carnivore diet is about exclusivity: consuming only animal products (especially meat) and avoiding any kind of plant foods altogether.

2. Stick To Three Meals A Day

When you start, it is advised to keep eating three meals a day or two meals and a snack - whatever your current routine is before starting the diet. That helps you spread out your meals evenly and include a larger quantity of food in your diet, which equals more protein and nutrients - components necessary for healing. This approach is particularly recommended for people trying to gain weight or those in a bulking phase at the gym.

If you're hitting the weights hard, you'll need to provide your muscles with a constant supply of amino acids and energy (calories). The highest quality amino acids come from animal foods, not plants. On the opposite side, if you want to maximize fat loss, you may additionally combine the carnivore diet with intermittent fasting (IF). You can achieve that by eating one or two meals a day with long periods of drinking just water (water fasting) or no water at all (dry fasting) in between.

3. Drink Bone Broth

If you get bored with drinking just water and no more sodas or energy drinks, then adding hot beverages, like various types of bone broth (from chicken, beef, lamb, etc) throughout the day is a good idea. Bone broth is the clear, protein-rich liquid obtained by simmering meaty joints and bones in water. Bone broth contains large amounts of collagen, a structural protein found in the skin, cartilage and bones of animals and humans.

When boiled, the collagen in connective tissue is broken down into gelatin and various other health-promoting amino acids, such as proline, hydroxyproline, glycine and glutamine.

Gelatine is the most abundant protein in bone broth. Once in the digestive tract, gelatin can bind with water to support the healthy transit of food through the intestines, alleviating constipation. Emerging scientific research also suggests that gelatin, alongside other amino acids found in bone broth, may have therapeutic potential in inflammatory bowel disease (IBD), such as ulcerative colitis and Crohn's disease.

4. Cook Meat To Desired Taste

When you first start the carnivore diet stick to the tastes and flavors that you normally like. If you happen to like your steak cooked rare, then you're already getting the most out of your food's nutritional value, as less cooking means less nutrients and enzymes being degraded by heat.

If you like your steak well-done, then stick with that temporarily and gradually move towards the rare side of things. Pork and poultry should always be cooked thoroughly and never eaten raw or rare. Raw chicken and pork can have bacteria that cause food poisoning including *Campylobacter*, *Salmonella*, *Clostridium perfringens* and *E. coli*. Symptoms of food poisoning may include fever, stomach cramping, diarrhea, and sometimes nausea and vomiting.

5. All Kinds Of Meat Are Your Friend

When you start following the carnivore diet, don't just head to your butcher and ask for pork chops and striploin steaks. Change things up between beef, pork, lamb, bison, buffalo, fresh fish, and even organ meats (offal). By switching things around on a daily basis, it allows you to maximize your intake of different types of nutrients (vitamins, minerals, trace elements, amino acids, etc.) preventing nutrient deficiencies. Plus, it keeps your diet rich and interesting.

6. Athletes Have To Be Patient For Results

High-performance athletes oftentimes struggle in the first couple of weeks of starting the carnivore diet. This is because their body no longer gets its energy from glucose, which is sourced from carbs. Instead, it now has to adapt to processing and utilizing more protein and fat.

Thus, a potential drop in energy isn't due to a lack of calories per se, but more so due to the type of calories their body now has to work with. Improvements in physical and mental energy and stamina will come, but for some athletes, adding some low-toxicity plant products (i.e., fruit) in the first couple of weeks can be helpful, just to keep their overall energy up to perform optimally.

How To Start The Carnivore Diet: Choose Your Level of Strictness

Making drastic changes to your diet can oftentimes be quite overwhelming. While the rules for carnivory are relatively simple, there are a few details to keep in mind if you want to get into this way of eating as smoothly as possible. For that reason, it is recommended to not go all in, but work your way up through different levels of strictness:

Level 1 (Introduction)

At level 1, the main rule is that if it's meat, it belongs to the plate. No stringent rules yet on the types of meat, cuts, or the level of processing.

At this level, you are allowed to enjoy beverages like tea, cocoa and coffee, and foods like eggs, full-fat cream, butter and cheese, just to give yourself a little diversity. Salt, pepper, some spices and electrolyte supplements are also allowed and will help make your food taste better.

Electrolyte supplements will reduce the negative side effects of any potential dehydration. This level may still seem like a big drastic change for some people, particularly those coming from the standard American diet (SAD). This introductory stage is meant to give you a better opportunity to physically and mentally prepare for the next, more strict stages.

Level 2 (Inflammation Buster)

After 2 to 4 weeks at level 1, you can take the next step and remove all non-meat products. From a dietary perspective, you'll be now taking in only meat, salt, water, and nothing else. You should also remove any highly processed meats like pastrami and salami, as well as dairy. Apart from salt and pepper, a few low-toxicity herbs and spices like oregano, thyme and rosemary, are also allowed, but avoid using them too much. The idea here is to take another big step towards joining true zero-carb carnivory.

Level 3 (Autoimmune Carnivore)

Once you've completed another 2 to 4 weeks at level 2, you can now move onto level 3, where the only allowable meat is red meat, such as beef, veal, goat, lamb, buffalo, venison, etc.

You can now switch between cuts as much as you like, and also get some organ meats (offal) as well, especially liver and spleen. This diet plan can become quite expensive, especially if you choose to go for organic, grass-fed meat only. If this lifestyle ends up becoming too costly, you may just stick to regular, non-organic red meat, preferably beef, veal or lamb, and avoid pork, fish and poultry as much as possible.

Level 4 (Relaxed Carnivore)

Stick with level 3 for about 30 days and start to observe the changes in your digestion, energy levels, mental health, body composition, and metabolism. We'll get to the benefits shortly, but most likely you will start noticing things such as increased physical and mental energy, improved mood and concentration, reduced pain and inflammation, and an overall upgrade in how you think, feel, look and perform. At level 4, it's time to slowly add in some of the things you removed in levels 2 and 3. Don't get this wrong though - you should still mainly focus on quality, grass-fed red meat, such as beef, veal, lamb or bison. It's just that having some regular new additions like fish, seafood, poultry and pork can help you to stay motivated. The aim of this stage is to identify the meat sources that make you feel bloated, sick, or unwell. Eventually, you should end up with a list of non-irritating animal foods to stick with long-term.

What Level To Choose?

Generally speaking, it is recommended that you start with level 1. But, if you're not a caffeine addict, you may also jump straight to level 2. Many people try to jump straight into level 3 and just struggle too much with all the restrictions it imposes.

Ideally, try to spend at least 30 days between levels 1 and 2 before you take that final step.

Mistakes To Avoid When First Starting The Carnivore Diet

1. Sneaking in small amounts of fruits and vegetables: Some people don't fully understand the meaning of carnivore and think that as long as their main source of food is meat, everything is fine. It's not fine. It's called the "carnivore diet" for a reason, so stick with animal products only.

2. Only buying lean cuts: Meat from all animals is available in lean and fatty cuts. You don't have to eat pork belly every day (pork belly is one of the fattiest cuts of meat), but don't be afraid of animal fat. Animal fat is what will provide your body with the fuel and nutrients it needs to thrive.

3. Drinking too little water: This is a problem for most Americans in general following any type of diet. However, since during carnivore you're eating a smaller volume of food, and most fruit and vegetables (that naturally contain plenty of water) are omitted, you'll have to consume more water than you normally would, ideally with some electrolytes such as potassium, sodium, magnesium, calcium and chloride. Plain water is a solvent (oftentimes called the "universal solvent") and doesn't contain any electrolytes. Thus, plain water doesn't hydrate you, but further dilutes your already existing electrolyte stores and makes you pee them out.

4. Not eating enough: The carnivore diet is not just about eating a little bit of meat here and there. You need to eat a decent amount of it, ideally, until you're full. Even if you are interested solely in weight loss, your body will need plenty of energy to keep going and keep your metabolic engine running.

5. Not adding salt: Electrolytes are vital for the salinity of your blood. When you eat just meat and no carbs or fiber, you may experience a reduction in your body's electrolyte levels. For that reason, you shouldn't be afraid to salt your meals liberally and even salt your water if you have to. Staying well-hydrated is very important for your mood, energy levels, digestive health, and more.

Carnivore Diet Benefits

1. Weight Loss

One of the biggest advantages of this diet is its ability to aid in weight loss. Many followers of the diet have found that it has helped them to lose weight when all other diets have failed them. Since you can eat as much as you want and as often as you want while on this diet, most carnivores rarely feel hungry. Additionally, the diet allows them to continue eating some of the foods that they love the most, such as steak and bacon.

The reason that the carnivore diet works so well for weight loss is that it eliminates high-carb, heavily processed ingredients, many of which are also high in calories. Decreasing your intake of these calorie-dense foods, such as chips, candy, crackers and cookies, helps promote weight loss and minimize inflammation in your body.

While clinical research on the carnivore diet specifically is limited, several studies have showcased that low-carb diets can prove particularly effective for weight loss. For example, a 2013 review published in the *British Journal of Nutrition* showed that following a very low-carb diet was able to boost long-term weight loss better in participants compared to a low-fat diet, suggesting that cutting carbs could be a useful strategy for combatting obesity.

2. Low in Added Sugars

Many of the foods not allowed on the carnivore diet are high in added sugars, including sugar-sweetened beverages, baked goods, candies and desserts. Added sugar can have a detrimental effect on nearly every aspect of health, with some research linking added sugar consumption to increased risk of obesity, heart disease, liver problems and even cancer.

Eliminating these foods from your diet could potentially reduce your risk of developing a chronic condition and improve future health outcomes if you already have one.

3. Rich in High-Quality Protein

Red meat, poultry, pork, fish and seafood and are key components of the carnivore diet, all of which are loaded with protein. Protein plays a central role in tissue repair, muscle building, growth and immune function. A protein deficiency can have serious consequences and may lead to symptoms such as hair loss, depression, weakness, vascular problems, stunted growth and anemia.

High-protein diets have been shown to enhance weight loss and reduce levels of ghrelin, one of the primary hormones that stimulate hunger. This helps to curb any cravings and keep your appetite in check. Ghrelin is a hormone that is produced and released mainly by the stomach with small amounts also released by the small intestine, pancreas and brain. It has numerous functions. It is termed the 'hunger hormone' because it stimulates appetite, increases food intake and promotes fat storage.

4. Reduces Inflammation

Chronic inflammation is one of the biggest culprits of the chronic disease pandemic we witness today. Obese people are particularly susceptible to the effects of chronic inflammation because excess fat tissue produces and secretes inflammatory molecules, such cytokines, which precipitate an inflammatory state in the body.

Chronic inflammation impairs brain and digestive function, and damages the vascular walls. For the last 50 years meat has been blamed for almost every ailment under the sun, including causing inflammation, when the real culprits are processed carbs and vegetables (seed) oils. A recent human study compared the standard low-fat, high-carb diet to a high-fat, low-carb diet in a group of obese adults. The results were the exact opposite of the common belief that a high-fat, low-carb diet is bad, showing far greater inflammation reductions in the test subjects following a high-fat, low-carb diet.

5. Improves Gut Health

If eating meat only makes your digestion feel better, that means you have an underlying gut issue (like most people in the Western world today). Many people with chronic digestive problems find great relief by adopting a carnivore diet, as it is a low-residue diet that limits difficult-to-digest, high-fiber foods such as whole grains, nuts, seeds, fruits, and vegetables. This starves potentially pathogenic bacteria and yeasts in the gut from their favorite food - carbs. The lack of fiber provides rest to the digestive system, which now doesn't have to work extra hard to process all this harsh plant material.

For this and other reasons, the carnivore diet is often prescribed to people suffering from inflammatory bowel disease (IBD) or irritable bowel syndrome (IBS), successfully eliminating negative symptoms such as gas, bloating, abdominal pain and diarrhea.

6. Helps You Identify Irritating Foods

The carnivore diet eliminates four of the seven most common food allergens: wheat, soy, peanuts (legumes), and tree nuts (almonds, walnuts, hazelnuts, pistachios, etc). Some strict variations of the diet may also eliminate eggs, dairy, fish and seafood. A strict all-meat, salt and water carnivore diet is, in essence, an extreme elimination diet that can prove very beneficial and even remedial for a big majority of chronic disease patients, particularly those dealing with chronic gut and autoimmune issues.

7. Enhances Cognition

Same as the ketogenic diet, the carnivore diet produces certain metabolic changes in your body, which now has to switch from using easily accessible glucose as fuel to fats and ketones. While many may think that glucose, an easily accessible form of energy, is a better fuel source for the brain than ketones, the opposite holds true.

One of the biggest challenges in relying on glucose as your primary fuel source is that you constantly go through fluctuations of peaks and troughs. Once you switch to ketones and fat, your body starts oxidizing these substrates which come either from your diet or your own fat reserves (i.e., love

45

handles, thighs, belly fat, etc). It's the ketones that give you that mental clarity and improved concentration when following a strict, low-carb carnivore diet.

It's worth noting though, that on many occasions an overly excessive protein intake can kick you out of ketosis by prompting your liver to produce glucose from amino acids through the process of gluconeogenesis. Thus, if you are particularly interested in staying in ketosis, you may need to follow a higher-fat, lower-protein carnivore diet variation, as well as use a ketone meter to regulate your ketone levels.

8. Helps Build Muscle

The number 1. ingredient for building muscle is a specific set of amino acids that comprise the building blocks of muscle protein in your body. It's impossible to build new muscle tissue without an excess of amino acids. People who struggle to eat enough meat, poultry, eggs, fish and dairy every day, oftentimes have to resort to dietary supplements, such as protein powders, in order to cover their needs for high-quality, bioavailable amino acids.

The carnivore diet naturally supplies your body with ample amounts of these anabolic amino acids that promote muscle protein synthesis (MPS). Muscle protein synthesis (MPS) is a naturally occurring process that occurs in your body where protein is produced to repair muscle damage caused by intense exercise. It is an opposing process to muscle protein breakdown (MPB) in which protein is lost as a result of exercise.

If MPS outpaces MPB, muscle growth manifests. Building new muscle indirectly helps with weight loss as increasing your muscle mass naturally raises your basic metabolic rate (BMR). That's because muscle tissue consumes more energy than fat/adipose tissue, making weight control easier and more sustainable.

Carnivore Diet Drawbacks

1. Carnivore "Flu"

Just like with the keto diet, when your body switches from using glucose to ketones, you go through an induction phase where you might feel like you have the flu. Stomach upset, aches and pains, and fatigue are all common and normal, but also temporary. Improvements come in a matter of days and these symptoms get fully reversed.

2. Nutrient Deficiencies

There are certain vitamins, like vitamin C, and minerals, such as potassium and magnesium, that are abundant in fruit and vegetables but in short supply in meat. Aside from that, the process of cooking food degrades some vitamins and minerals that are heat-sensitive (such as vitamin C and B), which means you'll always get less than the optimum amount when you overcook your food. One solution for this when following the carnivore diet is to use supplements like isolated vitamin complexes, multivitamins or mineral supplements.

The most common nutrient deficiencies that may manifest when following the carnivore diet for the long term include:

• **Vitamin C:** necessary as an antioxidant, collagen precursor, and for immune health.

• **Vitamin E:** necessary as an antioxidant, for immune and cardiovascular health.

• **Vitamin K:** necessary for blood clotting and calcium homeostasis.

• **Calcium:** necessary for bone density, oral health, nerve transmission, and muscle contractions.
• **Folate:** necessary for gene expression, cell replication and growth.
• **Magnesium:** necessary for enzyme activity, digestion, elimination, mineral/electrolyte balance and energy production.
• **Fiber:** important for metabolic stability, detoxification, colon health and microbiome diversity.
• **Phytonutrients:** necessary as antioxidants, substrates (food) for intestinal bacteria and detoxification processes.

3. Dehydration

In the first few days of following a strict all-meat carnivore diet, your body will eventually deplete all its glycogen reserves. Glycogen is a multibranched polysaccharide of glucose that serves as a form of energy storage. Glycogen represents the main storage form of glucose in the body and is made and stored primarily in the cells of the liver and skeletal muscles. Every molecule of glycogen binds to 3 parts of water.

At the beginning of your carnivore journey, as your glycogen stores will be getting depleted, that water will be released and processed by your kidneys. In just the first few days, you'll probably be going to lose about half a gallon of water. And this is just one pathway through which the carnivore diet can cause dehydration. There is another: high insulin levels in the body caused by eating carbs trigger your kidneys to hold onto water and sodium.

When you eliminate carbs and sugar from your diet altogether, your insulin levels drop, and your kidneys release this stored sodium and water. As water exits your body, you may find yourself getting thirsty. The same happens when you try the keto diet for the first time; it is a normal physiologic response that occurs when your diet suddenly lacks carbs and fiber.

This process alone can remove four to six pounds of water from your body. Along with the water, you will also lose lots of electrolytes, particularly sodium, potassium, calcium, magnesium and chloride, which will induce further dehydration.

CHAPTER 2: KETO VS CARNIVORE DIET

Many people get a little bit confused in telling the difference between a keto diet and a carnivore diet. After all, both diets restrict carbs and increase fat and protein-rich foods. Both in keto and carnivore, your body will be changing its metabolic style of functioning in a very similar fashion.

What Is The Keto Diet?

The ketogenic diet, or keto for short, is a low-carb, high-fat diet designed to switch your metabolism from glucose to ketones as a source of energy. The ketogenic diet has been around for a very long time and is not some new celebrity-endorsed idea with no proven track record through science. Keto was originally medically designed and clinically tested to help treat patients with epilepsy. The concept of keto is not all that difficult to understand, as it all comes down to how your body creates the raw energy your muscles and organs need to function. On a standard Western diet, you'll be loading up on carbs throughout the day, and these carbs would eventually get broken down and get converted into blood glucose.

Particularly when someone's diet is very high in sugar, this can lead to constant blood sugar spikes, which in the long-term may lead to serious health issues, including diseases like diabetes.

Keto, being very low-carb, aims to switch your metabolic style of function from carbs to fat and ketones (byproducts of fat metabolism). Minimizing your carb intake and relying primarily on dietary fat leads to the increased production of blood ketones, which now provide all the energy you need for daily activities and exercise.

The metabolic environment generated by a very low-carb, high-fat diet creates the ideal conditions for healthy, sustainable weight loss and reduced levels of inflammation in the body. Foods that the keto diet typically includes are the following:

• Meat
• Poultry
• Fish
• Seafood
• Eggs
• Low-lactose dairy (i.e., hard cheeses, cream, butter, full-fat yogurt)
• Low-carb vegetables (i.e., leafy greens, cruciferous vegetables, etc.)
• Low-carb fruit (i.e., avocados, olives, coconuts, melons, berries, etc.)
• Healthy fats and oils (i.e., olive oil, coconut oil, avocado oil, lard, tallow, duck fat, etc.)

What Is The Carnivore Diet?

As you probably already know, the carnivore diet is a high-fat, high-protein, low-carb diet that involves eating only meat with no plant foods whatsoever. Some dairy products, like raw milk, cheese and butter, as well as eggs, are oftentimes allowed depending on the carnivore diet variation.

The primary rule of the carnivore diet is to exclude all plant foods, which means you'll be cutting out 99% of the dietary sources of carbohydrates, pushing your body to start relying solely on protein and fats for its energy and calories. The carnivore diet typically includes the following foods:
• Red meat, especially the fattier cuts
• Poultry
• Fish and seafood
• Eggs
• Dairy
• Organ meats
• Bone broths
• Animal fats, such as lard and tallow

Some versions of the carnivore diet, such as the Lion Diet (includes ruminant meat, water and salt only), do not allow eggs and dairy. Some other less restrictive versions allow black coffee for those transitioning from a high-caffeine lifestyle. In general though, when following the carnivore diet all plant foods should be avoided, including:
• Grains
• Beans
• Fruits
• Vegetables
• Nuts and seeds
• Herbs and spices
• Alcohol
• Vegetable oils

Differences Between Keto and Carnivore

When it comes to the differences between keto and carnivore, it might seem obvious that in the carnivore diet, dieters eat only animal products with no plants whatsoever, while there is a little bit more flexibility in keto. Some details you should be aware of with regards to those diets, especially if you have no prior experience with them, include:

1. Keto Is More Flexible and Easier To Follow

On keto, you're allowed to consume some plant products and consequently carbs. For the average keto dieter, this will be somewhere around 50 grams of carbohydrates per day or lower. What this does is allow you to satisfy some of your food cravings, especially in the early days. It also gives you just that little bit more flexibility when it comes to your meal recipes to add some vegetables for more diversity and color.

And then there is fiber, which by and large is keto-friendly because it isn't counted as a net positive carb as most of it passes through your GI tract undigested. So, from a digestion and micronutrient perspective, there are some advantages that the keto diet may have over the carnivore diet. On the other hand, when following carnivore, all those plants and vegetables you may like are a no-go, which can make a lot of people feel pressured and fall of the wagon.

2. Cravings

When you switch your diet to animal products-only, you will be cutting out all carbs and increasing your fat and protein intake. Apart from meat, water, and bone broth (as well as eggs and dairy if you choose to include them), you won't be taking in anything else. For some people, this type of diet may seem like heaven, but it won't be long before you start craving some starchy veggies or even a small dessert from time to time.

If you've done keto, you may have experienced similar cravings while on it, but because carnivore prohibits all plant foods, your body may start interpreting this as a symptom of starvation. Thus, your brain and stomach can start sending your conscious signals that you need to eat other foods, and this can be quite a tough battle.

3. Meal Frequency

Some keto dieters like to spread out their food intake over four to six meals a day, depending on how many calories they're aiming for. They find that this approach helps limit feelings of hunger and reduces carb cravings, increasing adherence to the diet. However, the carnivore diet works a bit differently.

If you decide to follow a strict, meat-only carnivore diet, it's generally recommended to switch to three, and sometimes two meals a day. One reason for this is that most meat-only carnivore recipes usually involve just meat and butter or suet, and they don't taste that good when cold. Thus, for maximum enjoyment and palatability, it's recommended to prepare your meals fresh and eat them straight away. If you want to also include some intermittent fasting in your routine, you may skip breakfast altogether, which brings you close to a 14 - 16 hours fasting window.

4. Macronutrient Ratios

On the keto diet, the macronutrient ratios are typically 60% fat, 30% protein, and 10% carbs. What that 60/30/10 split means is that 60% of all your calories should come from healthy fats, with protein and carbs providing 30% and 10% of your total calories, respectively. That is a drastic shift from the 20-35% fats, 10-35% protein, 45-65% carbs ratio that conventional nutritional science recommends (according to the Institute of Medicine).

When it comes to the carnivore diet, there isn't one strict macronutrient ratio to keep to, as the diet is all about eating nutrient-dense, highly bioavailable animal products, especially meat. This means you'll only be ingesting animal protein and fat, with only a tiny, almost accidental, amount of carbs that can sneak in with some dairy products.

5. Need For Supplements

While both keto and carnivore limit the number of plant foods you can eat, there is some more flexibility to get the essential vitamins and minerals you need when following keto. This means that you may become a bit more reliant on supplements while on carnivore, or that you may need to add in some nutrient-dense organ meats (offal). Liver and spleen, for example, contain a wide variety of micronutrients in significant amounts that can help someone overcome serious, lifelong nutritional deficiencies. It's worth mentioning here that many keto supplements, bars, snacks and powders often contain more carbs than they should. So, be very cognizant when consuming these types of products as they can throw your metabolism off and lead to erratic shifts in blood glucose and ketone levels, amplifying the negative 'keto/carnivore flu' side effects.

Similarities Between Keto and Carnivore

The keto and carnivore diets have a lot of things in common, including side effects, metabolic changes, and health benefits. They are actually so closely related that many people switch between the two on a cyclical basis, especially after they have healed enough while doing carnivore.

1. Side Effects

The first similarity worth mentioning is the infamous 'keto/carnivore flu'. These are the flu-like symptoms of brain fog, muscle aches and pains, nausea, headaches, and fatigue that generally last for somewhere between 1 and 14 days. It's not a pleasant experience, but one of those hurdles you have to get over to enjoy all the healing, anti-inflammatory, and energy-boosting benefits that come with ketosis. The interesting thing is that when you switch from keto to carnivore, those symptoms may pop up again for a few days, so make sure you prepare properly for them.

Another common issue with both diets is bowel irregularity. One of the most commonly asked questions in forums and health websites is "does the keto diet cause constipation?" The answer is sometimes yes, sometimes no, and the same happens on the carnivore diet. This is often due to a lack of fiber, which is something that you may need to supplement with.

2. It's All About Fat

In both dietary approaches, there is a great emphasis on getting lots of healthy, quality fats from your diet. This would approximately amount to around 60 - 70% of your total daily energy intake, which is quite a lot. However, once your body switches to ketosis, all that extra fat will be converted into ketones (fuel). Ketones are a different form of energy than glucose that offer better cognitive performance and levels of alertness. Additionally, high amounts of fat are metabolized slower and don't pose a threat to your blood sugar health, particularly when you also follow a healthy exercise routine.

3. Metabolic Changes

On both keto and carnivore, your body will switch from glucose to ketones as its primary source of fuel. This metabolic adaptation is called 'ketosis' and is a vital function and feature of human evolution. Throughout human history, food and especially carbohydrates were not as abundant and available as they are today. There is a reason why historically people loaded up on carbs in the summer through fruits and vegetables, and then resorted to scarce animal products and stored body fat in the winter. Ketosis is a metabolic state that allows you to mobilize stored fat reserves that you don't need.

4. Weight Loss

As long as you calculate your calorie needs and stay below your daily threshold, you will trigger weight loss, whether you're on keto or carnivore or virtually any diet. By keeping your intake of dietary fat below what you need energy-wise, your body will go into starvation mode and use up all its glycogen and fat reserves. The results of this metabolic shift can be quite drastic, and as long as you faithfully stick to the guidelines of keto or carnivore, you will experience very steady, smooth and sustainable weight loss, which is the best type of weight loss.

5. Increased Physical And Mental Energy

One of the most significant benefits of ketosis, whether keto-induced or carnivore-induced, is that you will have a lot more readily available energy. And the nature of ketone-derived energy is that it doesn't regularly spike and fall as glucose does. As a result, you will perform better athletically and academically. For a big majority of people, it's exactly this mental clarity that makes them want to come back for more on keto or carnivore.

So, with all the keto-carnivore similarities explained, it's now time to discover how you can take advantage of both diets in a cyclical way.

Alternating Between Keto and Carnivore

While it is entirely possible to stick to a carnivore diet lifestyle long-term, it's worth admitting that at some point it may eventually become too strict and unsustainable for a lot of people. Especially around Thanksgiving or Christmas, but also when you head on vacation with friends, and you end up watching others enjoying all types of tasty food (pizza, fries, pasta, beer, wine, etc.) and all you can do is just sip on a glass of water or cup of bone broth. Sure, those summer BBQs are great, but there is a limit to the enjoyment.

A smart idea would be to cycle through phases of keto and carnivore. For example, you could do 6 to 10 weeks of nose-to-tail carnivore two or three times a year, and for the following time follow a very structured and clean ketogenic diet.

How To Transition From Keto To Carnivore

Ok, so let's assume you've done the keto diet thing and now you want to take it a step further and try the carnivore diet. How do you go about that? The answer lies in the following five simple and gradual steps:

1. Analyze Your Food Journal

If you don't already keep a food journal, then start immediately. You'll want to write down everything you eat so that you can see exactly how many calories you take in and what your macronutrient ratio is. What you may also do is print out your journal and then use a highlighting pen to mark all the animal foods you eat. This will give you a good idea of what percentage of your food actually comes from animals vs plants.

2. Calculate Your Calorie Intake From Plants

Now that you know how many calories you take in from meat and plants, you can determine how much you need to make up by replacing plants with animal products.

If you're at a healthy weight, then stick to the same number of calories while on the carnivore diet. If you have some way to go to reach your weight loss goals, then consider reducing your calories a little more.

Note that weight loss during an all-meat diet is more pronounced than on a ketogenic diet. Meat also tends to keep you full for longer, which means that you can reduce your calories more easily while on the carnivore diet.

3. Gradually Replace Greens With Meat

Every day for 7-10 days, simply remove any plant-based items from your diet and add in some more meat. This strategy makes it easier to transition from keto to carnivore. It also allows you to stick to the same exercise routine without having to worry too much about feeling drained or weak.

4. Diversify The Meats You Eat

Most people want some variety in their diet. One of the toughest things when following the carnivore diet is to constantly be eating the same stuff again and again. Even if it's a delicious ribeye steak or New York strip cooked in grass-fed butter, you can quickly get sick of it. To make your diet more enjoyable and interesting, the best thing you can do is switch between different types of meat - beef, lamb, bison, buffalo, pork, chicken, fish, and organ meats (offal). That strategy, on top of improving diet compliance, has the added benefit of providing you with a more diverse range of nutrients.

5. Monitor Your Ketone Levels

As you gradually reduce your carbohydrate intake and switch to more meat, you should notice an increase in ketone levels. You can buy devices and test strips that measure these levels in your urine reasonably accurately. Higher ketone levels are a good indicator that you're moving in the right direction. You should start testing them several times a day, keep track of the measures, and note down what kind of mood you're in. This may soon become a motivating task as generally speaking, you'll be in a better mood when your ketone levels are higher.

Keto vs Carnivore: Which Diet Is Better?

In the whole keto vs carnivore diet debate, it really shouldn't be a question of which one is better. These two diets are 'cousins' and complement each other. If you're new to dieting for health, it is recommended to start with keto first and then, after a few weeks start transitioning into carnivore with regular on and off cycles. Some people oftentimes ask "is simply going low-carb the same as keto or carnivore?" The answer is no, but if you are struggling to commit to any of these two lifestyles, then simply reducing your carb intake is a good start.

CHAPTER 3: VEGAN VS CARNIVORE DIET

Veganism is defined as a way of living that attempts to exclude all forms of animal exploitation and cruelty, whether for food, clothing, or any other purpose. Thus, a vegan diet is completely devoid of animal products, including meat, fish, seafood, eggs, and dairy. People may choose to follow a vegan diet for various reasons. These can range from ethics to environmental concerns, but they can also stem from a desire to improve health. Some vegan advocates believe that meat causes cancer and destroys the planet.

Meat-eaters, on the opposite hand, argue that animal foods are vitally important for human health and that giving up on them will lead to nutrient deficiencies and other health problems. Both sides propose that their approach is healthier and better than the other. If you put a group of vegans and carnivores in the same social media thread, one thing is nearly certain - they'll start arguing about food.

"Meat causes cancer!"

"You need meat for B12!"

"But meat production leads to climate change!"

"Meat-free processed food is just as bad!"

And on it will go.

What Is The Vegan Diet?

A vegan diet is a way of eating that eliminates all foods that come from an animal, including meat, fish, seafood, eggs and dairy products like milk, butter, cheese, and yogurt. Instead, people who follow the vegan diet eat plant-based foods, such as fruits, vegetables, nuts, seeds, beans and grains. Vegans oftentimes eat many of these plant foods raw. When a vegan diet is more than 80% raw, it's called a raw vegan diet.

Is The Vegan Diet Healthy?

A smartly designed plant-based (not vegan) diet can be healthy depending on the individual. Eating only whole, unprocessed plant-based foods and using supplements when necessary is an approach that can work well for a period of time, but may eventually lead to nutrient deficiencies. As with any diet, similarly, with veganism, it's all about how you follow a particular diet that determines if it will work or not.

Certainly, there are some benefits to eating a diet that is high in raw or lightly cooked foods, such as fruit and vegetables. When raw, these foods contain large amounts of enzymes that get otherwise lost during cooking or high-heat processing. Our body needs those enzymes to break these foods down into smaller, nutritional units that it can absorb and utilize.

According to many alternative medicine practices, such as natural hygiene (orthopathy) and TCM (traditional Chinese medicine), uncooked fruits and vegetables are biogenic or 'life-giving', while cooking them reduces their alkalinizing and healing properties. The therapeutic application of raw fruits and vegetables is a potential benefit of a plant-based diet that is rich

63

in raw, living foods. Additionally, consuming more greens, such as leafy greens and cruciferous vegetables, has been shown to help our body attain a normal pH, alkalizing and supporting its efforts towards homeostasis (balance).

A diet rich in whole fruits and vegetables has also been shown to be helpful in promoting a healthy response to inflammation, as well as supply the body with beneficial antioxidants and phytonutrients, such as polyphenols. Of course, with all those benefits come many potential pitfalls. For example, it's worth mentioning that while there have indeed been civilizations throughout history that have thrived on vegetarian diets, no tribe has ever flourished on a completely vegan diet, meaning a diet that excludes 100% of animal products. So, the word 'vegan' doesn't always mean that something is healthy. 'Vegan' is oftentimes an umbrella term used to describe diets comprised of highly processed plant foods and no animal products. A surprising amount of potato chips, cookies and candy bars are vegan. Does that mean that they are healthy? Absolutely not.

The most common theme on a vegan diet is not binge-eating chips or candy bars, but buying faux versions of meats and cheeses. We are not talking about fermented foods like tempeh or natto or even homemade vegan cheeses from nuts. We are talking about soy burgers, Tofurkey and the like, purchased at the grocery store. These foods are loaded with preservatives, table salt, sugar, gluten, soy and wheat. Unless such products are explicitly non-GMO, you can be almost certain you're ingesting some chemicals with your food.

If you ever try veganism, be very mindful of the amount of refined carbohydrates you are ingesting, such as pasta, crackers, biscuits and cereals. To be a healthy plant-based eater, skip all processed and packaged stuff, because these foods have been shown time and time again to promote weight gain, inflammation and metabolic damage. Instead, try to stick to a healthy version of a plant-based (not vegan) diet with lots of fresh, organic fruits, vegetables, nuts, seeds and the like.

Vegan Nutrient Deficiencies

To be healthy, vegetarians and especially vegans need to make sure they're getting enough protein, vitamin B12, vitamin D3, vitamin K2, calcium, iron, zinc and iodine among other nutrients. For example, The Academy of Nutrition and Dietetics warns of the risk of vitamin B12 deficiencies in vegetarians and vegans. Vitamin B12 is almost exclusively found in animal products.

The only plant foods that naturally contain trace amounts of bioactive vitamin B12 include Nori seaweed (a type of marine algae), tempeh (a fermented soy product) and Shiitake mushrooms. Nori seaweed is considered the most suitable source of biologically available B12 for vegans, though it doesn't provide a sufficient amount on its own. Raw or freeze-dried nori is superior to conventionally dried types. This is because some of the vitamin B12 is destroyed during the drying process.

However, all these vegan foods are not by any means sufficient sources of B12 and do not cover the daily requirements. Another plant food often claimed to contain vitamin B12 is spirulina, which offers only pseudovitamin B12, which is not biologically available, meaning it can't be absorbed and utilized by the body. For this reason, spirulina is unsuitable as a dietary source of vitamin B12. Practically, if someone wants to boost his/her vitamin B12 status without the use of dietary supplements, he/she needs to resort to animal products. This doesn't apply to just vitamin B12, but other nutrients as well. There are specific micronutrients that vegans can't get enough of or at all from their diet, no matter what they do:

1. Vitamin B12

Vitamin B12 is a crucial vitamin. It is needed for nerve tissue health, brain function, and the production of red blood cells. Another name for vitamin B12 is cobalamin. Deficiency in B12 results when its levels in the body are too low. That can lead to irreversible neurological damage. In the United States, as of 2021, between 1.5 and 15 percent of the population are diagnosed with vitamin B12 deficiency. Like all B vitamins, vitamin B12 is a water-soluble vitamin, meaning it can dissolve in water and travel through the bloodstream. The human body can store vitamin B12 for up to four years. Any excess or unwanted vitamin B12 is excreted in the urine. Vitamin B12 is the largest and most structurally complex vitamin. It occurs naturally in meat products and can only be industrially produced through bacterial fermentation synthesis.

Food Sources

Vitamin B12 is found naturally in animal foods, such as fish, meat, eggs, and dairy products. It does not typically occur in plant foods. To get sufficient amounts of vitamin B12, people following a vegan diet must supplement exogenously or eat foods that have been artificially fortified with it. These foods include:
• Enriched yeast extracts
• Soy products
• Breakfast cereals

• Bread
• Meat substitutes

Good dietary sources of natural, bioavailable B12 include:
• Beef
• Pork
• Ham
• Poultry
• Lamb
• Fish, especially haddock and tuna
• Dairy products, such as milk, cheese, and yogurt
• Eggs

Benefits

Vitamin B12 is crucial to the normal function of the brain and nervous system. It is also involved in the formation of red blood cells and helps create and regulate DNA. Metabolic processes taking place in every cell in the body depend on vitamin B12, as it plays a pivotal role in the synthesis of fatty acids and energy production.

Vitamin B12 enables the release of energy by helping the human body absorb folic acid (vitamin B9). Also, thanks to B12 the human body is able to produce millions of red blood cells every minute. These cells cannot multiply properly without vitamin B12. The production of red blood cells reduces when vitamin B12 levels are too low. Anemia may occur if the red blood cell count drops.

Intake Requirements

In the U.S., the National Institutes of Health (NIH) recommend that teens and adults over the age of 14 years should consume 2.4 micrograms (mcg) of vitamin B12 a day. Pregnant women should be sure to consume 2.6 mcg, and lactating women 2.8 mcg. Excessive intake of vitamin B12 has not demonstrated any toxic or harmful qualities. However, people are always advised to speak with their physician before starting to take B12 supplements. Some medications may interact with supplemental vitamin B12. These include metformin, proton pump inhibitors (PPIs), and h2 receptor agonists, often used for peptic ulcer disease. These drugs can interfere with vitamin B12 absorption. The antibiotic chloramphenicol (chloromycetin) may also interfere with red blood cell formation in people taking vitamin B12 supplements.

Deficiency

The symptoms and risks associated with vitamin B12 deficiency include:
• Weakness
• Fatigue
• Impaired brain function
• Sore mouth or tongue
• Weight loss
• Diarrhea
• Menstrual problems
• Increased susceptibility to infections
• Pale or yellowing skin
• Neurological disorders (including in babies of breastfeeding mothers)
• Psychiatric disorders

- Megaloblastic anemia
- Possible links to Alzheimer's disease
- Possible links to heart disease

2. Creatine

Creatine is a molecule found almost exclusively in animal foods. Most of it is stored in the muscles but significant amounts are also concentrated in the brain. It functions as an easily accessible energy reserve for muscle cells, giving them greater strength and endurance. For this reason, creatine monohydrate is one of the world's most popular and well-researched ergogenic supplements for muscle building. Studies show that creatine supplements can increase both muscle mass and strength.

Creatine is not a substance essential in the diet, since it can be produced by the liver. However, studies have shown that vegetarians and vegans tend to have lower levels of creatine in their muscles. One study, in particular, placed people on a lacto-ovo-vegetarian diet for 26 days and found that doing so caused a significant decrease in their muscle creatine levels.

Since creatine is naturally found in animal tissue, vegetarians and vegans can only get it from supplements, which is why for them creatine supplements may have more noticeable effects, including improvements in physical performance and brain function. For instance, vegetarians or vegans taking creatine supplements may experience significant improvements in their brain function while people who eat meat regularly may see no difference. This is attributed to the fact that meat-eaters already have higher levels of creatine in their muscles and brain due to their diet.

Food Sources

Best food sources of creatine include red meat and fish. One pound of raw beef or salmon provides 1 to 2 grams (g) of creatine.

Benefits

Creatine supplies chemical energy to parts of the body where it is needed in the form of ATP. Some of its benefits include:
• Improved athletic performance
• Increased body mass
• Enhanced recovery after exercise
• Antioxidant benefits
• Improved cognitive ability

Intake Requirements

A person needs between 1 and 3 grams (g) of creatine a day. Around half of this comes from diet, and the rest is synthesized by the body.

Deficiency

Creatine is a natural substance and essential for a range of body functions. An average young male weighing 70 kilograms (kg) has a store or pool of creatine of around 120 to 140 grams (g). This amount varies between individuals, and it depends partly on a person's muscle mass and their muscle fiber type composition (type I, type II, type III muscle fibers).

Around 95% of the creatine in the human body is stored in skeletal muscle, and 5% is in the brain. Between 1.5 and 2% of the body's creatine stores are converted for use each day by the liver, the kidneys, and the pancreas. Creatine deficiency is

linked to a wide range of conditions, including, but not limited to:
• Chronic obstructive pulmonary disease (COPD)
• Congestive heart failure (CHF)
• Depression
• Diabetes
• Multiple sclerosis (MS)
• Muscle atrophy
• Parkinson's disease
• Fibromyalgia
• Osteoarthritis

Oral creatine supplements or increasing dietary intake may relieve these conditions, but there is not yet enough evidence to prove that this is an effective treatment for most of them. Supplements can also be taken to increase creatine in the brain. This may help relieve seizures, symptoms of autism, and movement disorders, such as restless leg syndrome.

3. Carnosine

Carnosine is an antioxidant that's concentrated in the muscles and brain of humans and animals. It's very important for muscle function, and high levels of carnosine in muscles are linked to reduced muscle fatigue and improved athletic performance.

Carnosine is only found in animal foods. However, it's considered non-essential, since the body can form it from the amino acids histidine and beta-alanine. Dietary sources of beta-alanine may contribute to muscle levels of carnosine, but the main dietary sources - meat, poultry, and fish - are neither vegan nor vegetarian. Studies have shown that vegetarians and vegans have less carnosine in their muscles than meat-eaters.

Food Sources
The top food sources of carnosine are meats, such as turkey, chicken, beef, or pork. Other animal products such as eggs, milk, and cheese contain carnosine, but only in trace amounts. Since carnosine is found in large amounts in muscle tissue, the higher its concentration, the stronger that muscle will be. Unfortunately, contemporary industrial farming methods tend to prioritize fattening over muscle-building of animals raised for meat. Therefore, most modern food sources do not contain optimal amounts of carnosine.

Benefits
Some of carnosine's health benefits include:
• Improved mental acuity and cognitive function
• Increased muscle strength and endurance
• Cardiovascular support
• Antioxidant benefits
• Improved bone health

Intake Requirements
There's no agreement as to what dosage of carnosine will produce therapeutic effects. The appropriate dose of carnosine depends on several factors such as the person's age, health, and several other conditions. Among proponents, the recommended dosage ranges from 150 milligrams a day to around 1,000 milligrams a day.

Deficiency
Neurological disorders associated with carnosine deficiency, and the resulting carnosinemia (carnosine in the blood) may occur when deficiency is present. During carnosinemia, an

excess of carnosine in the urine, cerebrospinal fluid, blood, and nervous tissue cause a variety of neurological symptoms. These may include hypotonia (decreased muscle tone), developmental delays, mental retardation, nerve degeneration, sensory neuropathy, tremors, and seizures.

4. Vitamin D3 (Cholecalciferol)

Vitamin D is an essential nutrient/prohormone with many important functions in the human body. It plays an essential role in calcium and phosphorus homeostasis, and bone metabolism. Also called the 'sunshine vitamin', vitamin D doesn't come from diet alone. Your skin can synthesize vitamin D when it's exposed to sunlight. However, if your sunlight exposure is limited or you live far from the equator, you must get it from food or supplements. Deficiency in vitamin D is linked to an increased risk of various adverse conditions, including:

• Osteoporosis, with an increased risk of fractures in older adults
• Cancer
• Heart disease
• Multiple sclerosis
• Depression
• Impaired brain function
• Muscle wasting and reduced strength, especially in older adults
• Autoimmune disease

Food Sources

There are two types of dietary vitamin D:
• Ergocalciferol (D2), found in plants.
• Cholecalciferol (D3), found in animal foods.

Of these types, cholecalciferol (D3) increases blood levels of absorbable vitamin D much more efficiently than ergocalciferol (D2). The best sources of vitamin D3 are fatty fish and egg yolks. Other sources include supplements, cod liver oil, or enriched foods like milk or cereals. Since the main dietary sources of vitamin D3 are not plant-based, vegetarians and vegans are at a higher risk of deficiency, especially during the winter in countries north or south of the equator.

Benefits

Vitamin D has a wide range of health benefits. More specifically, it:
• Supports the immune system and fights disease
• Improves calcium metabolism
• Increases bone mineral density
• Reduces risk of osteoporosis
• Increases energy production
• Boosts weight loss
• Reduces depression

Intake Requirements

How much vitamin D you need depends on many factors, such as:
• Age
• Ethnicity
• Latitude
• Season

• Sun exposure
• Clothing
This is only a partial list of factors that can help determine the amount of vitamin D a person needs. The National Institutes of Health (NIH) recommend an average daily intake of 400 – 800 IU, or 10–20 micrograms (mcg). However, some studies find the daily intake needs to be much higher, particularly if you aren't being exposed to the sun or have a darker skin tone. Depending on who you ask, blood levels above 20 ng/ml or 30 ng/ml are considered sufficient.

One study involving healthy adults showed that a daily intake of 1,120 - 1,680 IU of vitamin D was needed to maintain sufficient blood levels. In the same study, individuals who were vitamin D deficient needed 5,000 IU to reach blood levels above 30 ng/ml. Studies in postmenopausal women with vitamin D levels below 20 ng/ml found that ingesting 800 – 2,000 IU of vitamin D raised blood levels above 20 ng/ml.

However, higher doses were needed to reach 30 ng/ml. People who are overweight or have obesity may also need higher amounts of vitamin D. All things considered, a daily vitamin D intake of 1,000–5,000 IU, or 25–125 micrograms (mcg), should be enough to ensure optimal blood levels in most people.

Deficiency

Vitamin D deficiency is a problem in most countries of the world. It's more pervasive in young women, infants, older adults, and people who have dark skin. About 42% of the U.S. population is vitamin D deficient. This rate rises to 82% in black people and 70% in Hispanics, which systemic problems likely play a role in. If you have access to strong sun all year, then occasional sun exposure may be enough to fulfill your

vitamin D requirements. However, if you live far north or south of the equator, your vitamin D levels may fluctuate depending on the season. These levels may go down during the winter months due to a lack of sufficient sunlight. In that case, you may need to rely on your diet or supplements for vitamin D as well as on the vitamin D that's stored in your body fat. In adults, a vitamin D deficiency may:
• Cause muscle weakness
• Intensify bone loss
• Increase the risk of fractures
• Impair immune function
In children, a severe vitamin D deficiency can cause delays in growth and rickets (a disease where the bones become soft). Furthermore, vitamin D deficiency is linked with several cancers, type 1 diabetes, multiple sclerosis (MS), high blood pressure, and thyroid problems.

5. Docosahexaenoic Acid (DHA)

Docosahexaenoic acid or DHA is an essential omega-3 fatty acid that's important for normal brain development and function. Deficiency in DHA can have adverse effects on mental health and brain function, especially in children. In addition, inadequate DHA intake in pregnant women may adversely affect fetal brain development.

Food Sources

It's mainly found in fatty fish, fish oil, and certain types of microalgae. In the body, DHA can also be made from the conversion of the omega-3 fatty acid alpha-linolenic acid (ALA), which is found in high amounts in flax seeds, chia seeds, and walnuts. However, the conversion of ALA to DHA is very inefficient and may not increase blood levels of DHA sufficiently. For this reason, vegetarians and vegans typically have lower levels of DHA than meat-eaters.

Benefits
Some of the benefits of DHA include:
• Suppressed inflammation
• Reduced heart disease risk
• Improvements in ADHD symptoms
• Reduced risk of early preterm births
• Accelerated muscle recovery after exercise
• Support of age-related macular degeneration, dry eyes, and diabetic eye disease (retinopathy)
• Lowered risk of several types of cancer, including colorectal, pancreatic, breast, and prostate cancer
• Nervous system health
• Prevention or slowing in the progress of Alzheimer's disease
• Lowered blood pressure
• Improved blood circulation
• Normal brain and eye development in babies
• Men's reproductive health support
• Healthy neurotransmitters and improved mood

Intake Requirements
To date, there is no official recommended daily allowance (RDA) for DHA. However, most health organizations agree that 250 – 500 mg of combined EPA and DHA is enough for adults to maintain good health. Higher amounts up to 4 grams are often recommended for certain health conditions. Dietary omega-6 intake affects someone's omega-3 needs, including DHA.

The typical Western diet contains around 10 times more omega-6s than omega-3s. These omega-6 fatty acids, such as canola oil, cottonseed oil, sunflower oil, safflower oil, soybean oil, etc, come mainly from refined vegetable (seed) oils that are added to processed food. Many experts believe that the optimal omega-6 to omega-3 ratio is about 2:1 or 1:1. Omega-6s and omega-3s compete for the same enzymes, which convert the fatty acids into their biologically active forms.

Therefore, if you wish to improve your omega-3 status, you should not only ensure an adequate intake of omega-3s from your diet and/or supplements, but also consider minimizing your total intake of vegetable (seed) oils and processed foods high in omega-6s.

Deficiency

It's important to ensure adequate consumption of omega-3 fatty acids, EPA and DHA, every day. These fatty acids are an important component of your cell membranes. Your body also needs them to produce signaling molecules called eicosanoids, which help your immune, pulmonary, cardiovascular, and endocrine systems work properly. Currently, there is no standard test to diagnose an omega-3 deficiency, though there are several ways to analyze omega-3 levels. Among many potential symptoms, these are some primary signs that you may be deficient in the omega 3 fatty acids EPA and DHA:

• Depression and/or anxiety
• Dry eyes
• Joint pain and stiffness
• Skin irritation and dryness
• Hair changes

6. Heme Iron

Heme iron is a type of iron found only in animal products, especially red meat. It's much better absorbed than non-heme iron, another form of iron commonly found in plant foods. Heme iron improves the absorption of non-heme iron from plant foods. This phenomenon is not entirely understood, but it is called the "meat factor."

Non-heme iron is generally poorly absorbed. Its absorption is further limited by anti-nutrients present in plant foods, such as phytic acid. Unlike non-heme iron, the absorption of heme iron is not affected by the presence of anti-nutrients. For this reason, vegetarians and vegans — especially females and people on raw food diets — are more prone to anemia than meat-eaters.

Food Sources

In the human diet, the primary sources of heme iron are the haemoglobin and myoglobin from consumption of meat, poultry, and fish whereas non-heme iron is obtained from cereals, pulses, legumes, fruits, and vegetables. The average absorption of heme iron from meat-containing meals is about 25 percent. The absorption of heme iron can vary from about 40 percent during iron deficiency to about 10 percent during iron repletion. Heme iron can be degraded and converted to non-heme iron if foods are cooked at a high temperature for too long. Calcium is the only dietary factor that negatively influences the absorption of heme iron and does so to the same extent that it influences non-heme iron. The greatest dietary sources of heme iron include:

• Oysters, clams, mussels
• Beef or chicken liver
• Organ meats

- Sardines
- Beef
- Poultry
- Tuna

Benefits

Iron helps to preserve many vital functions in the human body, including general energy and focus, gastrointestinal processes, immune function, red blood cell formation, and the regulation of body temperature. The benefits of iron often go unnoticed until a person is not getting enough. Iron deficiency anemia, which refers to a lack of adequate healthy red blood cells in the blood, can cause symptoms of fatigue, heart palpitations, pale skin, and breathlessness. Some of the benefits of heme iron include:

- Increased energy
- Improved delivery of oxygen to tissues and cells
- Better athletic performance
- Better immunity
- Lowered risk of premature birth
- Lowered risk of low birth weight
- Reduced irritability and better mood
- Reduced susceptibility to infections

Intake Requirements

Iron functions as a component of a number of proteins, including enzymes and hemoglobin, the latter being important for the transport of oxygen to tissues throughout the body for metabolism. Almost two-thirds of iron in the body is found in hemoglobin present in circulating erythrocytes. A readily mobilizable iron store contains another 25 percent. Most of the remaining 15 percent is in the myoglobin of muscle tissue and a variety of enzymes necessary for oxidative metabolism and many other functions in all cells. A 75-kg adult man contains about 4 grams of iron (50 mg/kg), while a menstruating woman has about 40 mg/kg of iron because of her smaller erythrocyte mass and iron storage. The Recommended Daily Allowance (RDA) for elemental iron depends on a person's age and sex. Elemental iron refers to the total amount of iron released from its bound form in food or supplements:

Infants
- 0 to 6 months: 0.27 milligrams (mg)
- 7 to 12 months: 11 mg

Children
- 1 to 3 years: 7 mg
- 4 to 8 years: 10 mg

Males
- 9 to 13 years: 8 mg
- 14 to 18 years: 11 mg
- 19 years and older: 8 mg

Females
- 9 to 13 years: 8 mg
- 14 to 18 years: 15 mg
- 19 to 50 years: 18 mg
- 51 years and older: 8 mg
- During pregnancy: 27 mg
- When lactating between 14 and 18 years of age: 10 mg
- When lactating at older than 19 years: 9 mg

Deficiency

Iron deficiency anemia is a common type of anemia — a condition in which blood lacks adequate healthy red blood cells (erythrocytes). Red blood cells carry oxygen to the body's tissues. As the name implies, iron deficiency anemia is due to insufficient iron. Without enough iron, your body can't produce enough of a substance in red blood cells that enables them to carry oxygen (hemoglobin). As a result, iron deficiency anemia may leave you tired and short of breath. You can correct iron deficiency anemia through diet or with iron supplementation. Iron deficiency anemia signs and symptoms include:

• Extreme fatigue
• Weakness
• Pale skin
• Chest pain
• Fast heartbeat
• Shortness of breath
• Headache, dizziness, or lightheadedness
• Cold hands and feet
• Inflammation or soreness of the tongue
• Hair loss
• Brittle nails
• Sensitivity to cold
• Confusion, loss of concentration
• Pica: cravings for dirt, clay, ice, or other non-food items

7. Taurine

Taurine is a sulfur compound found in various body tissues, including your brain, heart, and kidneys. While its bodily function is not entirely clear, it appears to play a role in muscle function, bile salt formation, and antioxidant defenses. Taurine is found only in animal-sourced foods, such as fish, seafood, meat, poultry, and dairy products. Subsequently, studies have shown that vegans have lower levels of taurine than meat-eaters. Your body can make much of the taurine it needs, but you need more from your diet to support the function of amino acids (amino acids are organic compounds that make proteins). Research shows that getting extra taurine from your diet confers other health benefits and may even be required for people with certain health conditions.

Food Sources
The best natural dietary sources of taurine include:
• Shellfish, especially scallops, clams, and mussels
• Tuna
• Tilapia
• Octopus
• Turkey
• Chicken
• Beef

Benefits
Some of the health benefits of taurine include:
• Lowered risk of diabetes
• Better blood sugar regulation
• Improved cardiovascular health

- Improved cholesterol and triglyceride levels
- Better arterial elasticity
- Normalized blood pressure
- Antioxidant protection
- Enhanced muscle recovery
- Improved muscle strength
- Increased stamina and endurance
- Increased metabolism

Intake Requirements

On average, most people consume about 400 milligrams of taurine per day in their diet. Studies that point to potential health benefits require much higher doses and show that getting up to 3,000 milligrams per day is safe.

Deficiency

Taurine serves a wide variety of functions in the central nervous system (CNS) - from development to cytoprotection, and taurine deficiency is associated with:
- Cardiomyopathy
- Renal dysfunction
- Developmental abnormalities
- Severe damage to retinal neurons (nerve cells that innervate the retina)

8. Vitamin K2

Vitamin K helps with blood clotting and wound healing. There are two types of vitamin K: vitamin K1 (phylloquinone) and vitamin K2 (which has several subtypes called menaquinones, known by the acronym 'MK'). Vitamin K1 occurs naturally in many plants, especially dark, leafy greens.

Vitamin K2 is present in some dairy products and egg yolks. Since vegans exclude dairy and eggs, they should focus on consuming the other dietary source of vitamin K2, which is fermented foods. Examples of vegan-friendly fermented foods that may contain vitamin K2 include:

• Raw sauerkraut
• Natto, a fermented soybean dish
• Unpasteurized kombucha
• Vegan kimchi
• Plant-based kefir

Many vegans end up deficient in vitamin K2, given that our gut bacteria are the ones that turn vitamin K1 from food into vitamin K2. Dysbiosis, chronic latent infections, and many other factors may render someone unable to convert ingested vitamin K1 from plants to vitamin K2 efficiently.

Many vegans require vitamin K2 supplementation in order to prevent future health complications associated with vitamin K2 deficiency, such as osteoporosis, low bone mineral density, and soft tissue calcification.

Food Sources

Good dietary sources of vitamin K2 include:
• Dairy products, especially hard cheeses
• Liver and other organ meats
• Beef
• Pork
• Egg yolks
• Chicken
• Fatty fish, such as salmon

Benefits

Some of the benefits of vitamin K2 include:
• Improved calcium homeostasis
• Strong bones and teeth
• Prevention of soft tissue calcification
• Improved cardiovascular health
• Healthy blood clotting
• Anticancer benefits

Intake Requirements

The Office of Dietary Supplements (ODS) recommends a daily intake of 120 micrograms (mcg) of vitamin K for adult males and 90 mcg for adult females. There is no specific recommendation for vitamin K2 (menaquinone) over vitamin K1 (phylloquinone).

Deficiency

Newborns and people with certain gastrointestinal disorders, such as Celiac disease and ulcerative colitis (UC), have a higher risk of vitamin K deficiency. A severe deficiency increases the time it takes for blood to clot, making a person more prone to bruising and bleeding and increasing the risk of hemorrhage.

A deficiency of the vitamin also reduces bone mineralization, which can lead to osteopenia and osteoporosis. Certain medications can affect vitamin K levels in the body. For example, long courses of antibiotics can kill the beneficial bacteria that convert vitamin K1 to vitamin K2.

Some cholesterol-lowering medications can also interfere with the body's ability to absorb vitamin K. Blood thinners, such as warfarin, may also interact dangerously with vitamin K supplements.

9. Zinc

Zinc is a nutrient that plays many vital roles in the human body. Because our body can't produce zinc on its own, we must obtain it through food or supplements. Zinc helps our immune system and metabolism function. It is also important for wound healing and our sense of taste and smell.

Zinc is naturally found in a wide range of plant and animal foods. For example, there are some plant-based sources like legumes, nuts, seeds, oats, and tofu, that contain good amounts of zinc. However, plant compounds called phytates, which occur in many legumes and cereals, impair its absorption. While not all vegans have low zinc intake, a 2013 systematic review and meta-analysis noted that vegans and vegetarians tend to have lower overall zinc levels compared to meat-eaters.

Food Sources
The best dietary sources of zinc include:
• Meat
• Poultry
• Shellfish
• Organ meats
• Dairy
• Eggs

Benefits
Zinc is required for numerous processes in our body, including:
• Gene expression

- Enzymatic reactions
- Immune function
- Protein synthesis
- DNA synthesis
- Wound healing
- Growth and development
- Thyroid hormone metabolism
- Androgen production

Intake Requirements

The recommended daily amount (RDA) of zinc is 8 milligrams (mg) for women and 11 mg for adult men.

Deficiency

Zinc is used by your body in cell production and immune processes. Although there is still a lot more to learn about zinc, we do know that it is an essential part of growth, sexual development, and reproduction. When you're zinc deficient, your body can't produce healthy, new cells. This leads to symptoms such as:

- Unexplained weight loss
- Wounds that won't heal
- Lack of alertness
- Decreased sense of smell and taste
- Diarrhea
- Loss of appetite
- Open sores on the skin

What Do the Vegan and Carnivore Diets Have in Common?

There are some nutrition fundamentals that most health-focused diets, including vegan and carnivore, focus on. Typically, these diets encourage their followers to:

- Emphasize whole foods
- Get enough quality protein
- Avoid foods rich in omega-6s (pro-inflammatory)
- Prioritize high nutrient density
- Chew well and eat until satisfied
- Minimize processed foods
- Go organic, when possible

CHAPTER 4: CARNIVORE DIET AND AUTOIMMUNITY

One of the reasons that the carnivore diet was brought into the spotlight in the first place was its ability to reduce or even reverse autoimmune symptoms. In this chapter, we've broken down how and why the carnivore diet can help with the management and/or reversal of various autoimmune conditions. So far, anecdotal reports from all over the world have showcased phenomenal results with regards to the benefits of the carnivore diet on autoimmunity. Lifelong autoimmune sufferers are able to achieve remission and notice their symptoms and pain go away. Contrary to the popular belief of eating your vegetables to stay healthy, eating a highly plant-based diet is not always the best approach when dealing with a complex, chronic health issue, such as autoimmune conditions.

Why Does The Carnivore Diet Work So Well For Autoimmunity?

There are many reasons that the carnivore diet helps with autoimmune disease and has to do with two primary factors that greatly increase someone's chance of getting an autoimmune condition:

• Chronic nutrient deficiencies (protein, health fats, vitamins, minerals, trace elements, enzymes, etc.)

• Toxicity from various sources (food, water, EMFs, environmental toxicity, geopathic stress, mold toxicity, heavy metals, etc.)

If you have an autoimmune condition, the carnivore diet may help you restore your health for several reasons:

1. It Eliminates Synthetic Additives and Processed Sugar

In the last 50 years, the mass production of processed foods increased exponentially. If you go to the supermarket today, most isles are filled with something that is packed or processed. And there lies a big problem: to make these foods convenient, palatable and long-lived, there is a whole slew of synthetic substances that must be added to them. To be sure these foods sell, food companies make them taste great, have a long shelf life, improve their consistency and texture, and most importantly - be cheap and available to all socioeconomic classes.

There is though one big price to pay. Some people, seems like more and more, have guts that can't handle these man-made additives added to these foods. Many of these substances interact with our gut lining, weakening it, and over time create inflammation and cause the so-called leaky gut syndrome. Leaky gut or gut permeability essentially means that toxins, undigested food particles, bacteria and viruses are able to pass into the bloodstream, where under healthy conditions they should never be. When this phenomenon occurs it triggers a response from your immune system, causing immune cell migration to various parts of your body (inflammation) and especially where you are genetically predisposed to (colon, thyroid, joints, skin, etc).

91

By nature, inflammation is a normal and healthy response from your immune system in order to clear contamination from your tissues. However, when a leaky gut allows substances to constantly pass into your bloodstream and contamination occurs on a regular basis, the results are chronic inflammation and immune excitation, which add up over time. After some time, which is different for everyone, the immune system gets dysregulated and that's when you get an official diagnosis of an autoimmune condition. In complete opposition to that scenario, when you switch to a meat-only carnivore diet, all synthetic additives are eliminated and your body has finally the strength, energy and resources it needs to rebuild that essential gut barrier.

That's why it's recommended that followers of the carnivore diet should eat only unprocessed, high-quality meat that is minimally spiced and ideally prepared at home. In that way, you are in total control of what goes into your food and ensure that your immune system doesn't get constantly 'poked' by harmful, irritating substances.

2. It Improves Gut Health

The health status of our gut is deeply connected to the health status of our microbiome. The microbiome is the aggregation of the genetic material of all bacteria, fungi, protozoa and viruses that live on and inside our body. Put simply, our overall health is not solely dictated by your human components. Our bodies harbor a huge array of microorganisms.

Bacteria are the biggest players, but we also host other single-celled organisms known as archaea, as well as fungi, viruses and other microbes, including viruses that attack bacteria. Together these are dubbed the human microbiota or microbiome. Some of these microorganisms are pathogens, but others only become harmful if they get in the wrong place or boom in number. Some others though are useful to our body because they help it break down food and absorb nutrients, as well as produce their own vital nutrients. B complex vitamins and vitamin K2 are vitamins that, in normal conditions, our gut bacteria produce.

Our gut microbiome is the equivalent of 2 - 3 lbs of bacteria and other microorganisms that exist in our gut. The carnivore diet has been shown to help correct a disrupted microbiome (called dysbiosis) by starving off many of the 'bad guys', which love to feast on simple sugars and processed carbohydrates. This is a huge step in returning your gut health back to a state of homeostasis and proper functionality.

Since a strict carnivore diet contains virtually no fiber, your gut will stop cultivating certain kinds of bacteria that thrive on dietary fiber. Now, you may disagree and say "I thought we needed fiber to be healthy!" Well, the answer depends on the context. Remember, dysbiosis is when the ratios of specific bacterial strains are flipped. That means that adding dietary fiber can exacerbate that imbalance. For people who have bad ratios of bacteria in their gut (dysbiosis), avoiding dietary fiber can oftentimes prove very beneficial, and facilitate gut healing, alleviating chronic digestive issues, such as gas, bloating, indigestion, constipation, and more.

3. It Is Very Nutrient-Dense and Anti-Inflammatory

Meat, fish, seafood, eggs, poultry and dairy are excellent sources of protein and essential fatty acids. They also constitute great sources of a host of other nutrients that our body needs to function optimally and stay healthy, such as iodine, heme iron, zinc, copper, B vitamins (especially B12), potassium, sodium, magnesium, calcium, taurine, carnitine, creatine, omega-3s (EPA and DHA) and cholesterol.

By default, animal products contain large amounts of bioavailable protein (protein that our body can actually absorb and utilize), which is vital for proper immune function (antibodies are proteins at the end of the day), tissue repair, growth and development.

Some of the most important nutrients present in animal products include:

• Iodine and L-tyrosine to help our body produce thyroid hormones.

• Iron to carry oxygen around our body.

• Zinc to keep our immune system strong, our skin healthy, and for growth, development, and reproductive health.

• Vitamin B12 for nervous system health, blood health, and energy production.

• Omega-3s to support our heart, brain, and nervous system, as well as keeping inflammation and triglycerides levels low.

• Cholesterol to assist our sex organs and adrenal glands in producing androgens, estrogens and corticosteroids.

• Vitamin D3 (cholecalciferol), which is essential for calcium and phosphorus homeostasis, as well as regulating (calming or stimulating) our immune system.

• Taurine to support muscle function, bile salt formation, and our antioxidant defenses.

4. Plants Don't Want To Be Eaten

All life forms on earth have powerful, innate adaptive mechanisms that increase their chance of survival and replication. Plants are no exception. To defend themselves against herbivores, plants have evolved through time to be masters of biochemical warfare. They carry incredibly sophisticated defense mechanisms (morphological, biochemical, and molecular) to counter the effects of herbivore attacks.

Their biochemical mechanisms of defense against herbivores are wide-ranging, highly dynamic, and mediated by both direct and indirect defenses. They produce plant defensive compounds either constitutively or in response to plant damage, and these compounds affect the feeding, growth, and survival of herbivores. In addition, to defend themselves, plants release volatile organic compounds (VOCs) that attract the natural enemies of herbivores. All these defense strategies act either independently or in conjunction with each other. Our understanding of these plant defensive mechanisms is still surprisingly limited, primarily due to their complexity.

A few of the many well-known plant defense chemical compounds that play a potential role in autoimmunity are lectins (including prolamins, such as gluten, and agglutinins, like wheat germ agglutinin), oxalates, phytates, saponins, and alkaloids. These are all plant toxins contained in many plant-based foods that are considered 'healthy' by most people. If you think about it, it makes sense: since plants can't attack or escape from their predators as animals do, they specialize in making biochemicals that cause digestive distress, infertility, or even death to the animals that attack them.

Now you may think "but we've been eating plants for millennia. Why all of a sudden do these plants cause us immune and digestive problems?" There are a few explanations and points to consider here:

• We never ate food that had that many synthetic additives and agrochemicals as it has today.

• We never made plants to be the basis of our human nutrition or replacement for animal foods.

• Our ancestors always prepared plant foods thoroughly before consuming them: they soaked, sprouted, fermented and/or cooked them to deactivate/remove plant toxins and increase their nutritional value, digestibility and bioavailability. Salads and raw vegetables weren't the most appreciated foods amongst our predecessors.

• Processed sugar and refined carbohydrates weren't available.

• Fruits and vegetables were eaten seasonally, not all year.

• Seed (vegetable) oils didn't exist and weren't part of the human diet.

• Breastfeeding babies for extended periods was the norm and ensured that the newborn was able to cultivate a healthy and diverse microbiome and immune system. The denatured powder baby formulas of today didn't exist.

• These days we breed and cultivate plants that are genetically engineered (GMOs) and more and more resistant to pesticides, hence more toxic to our body. Modern crops are sprayed heavier than in the past because the plants' DNA is altered to withstand heavier agrochemical baths.

The radical technological advancements that took place in the last 100 years in the food industry, biotechnology, and agricultural business destroyed our health and overall adaptability. The accumulation of those and many other factors decreased our tolerance to various types of stressors, rendering our gastrointestinal systems dysfunctional and 'leaky', allowing plant toxins and other normally tolerable compounds to infiltrate our bloodstream and chronically stimulate our immune system.

If it wasn't for all those changes, our guts would have been much more resilient and capable of tolerating plant defense compounds, such as anti-nutrients. We would be able to digest these foods much better and assimilate their nutrients better, withstanding any potential gastrointestinal irritations. Put simply, plant toxins are not the primary etiological factor in autoimmunity. They just exacerbate an already dysfunctional and imbalanced system.

CHAPTER 5: CARNIVORE DIET RECIPES

The best way to follow any diet in the long term is to actually enjoy it. Making sure that you cook meals that taste great and make you feel happy and satisfied will help you stay consistent and enjoy the amazing benefits of the carnivore diet. To help you with that, we have prepared some amazing carnivore recipes you may execute - no matter your level - at the comfort of your own home. Some things to keep in mind though: if you are battling an autoimmune condition or trying to minimize inflammation as much as possible, skip all recipes that include dairy, eggs, and processed meats, such as cured meats.

A strict carnivore elimination diet consisting of only 3 ingredients - ruminant meat (i.e., beef, lamb, buffalo, etc.), salt and water is a great, safe and effective way to get out of an autoimmune flare fast and start feeling great again. So, enjoy these delicious recipes and when necessary, don't hesitate to modify a few things to match your individual tastes and preferences!

Snacks & Appetizers

Hard-Boiled Eggs
Cook Time: 12 mins
Total Time: 12 mins

Yield: 6 to 12 eggs

Ingredients
• 6 to 12 large pasture-raised eggs

Instructions
1. Cover the eggs in a saucepan with water. Fill a saucepan about a quarter of the way with cold water. Place the eggs in a single layer at the bottom of the saucepan. Add more water so that the eggs are covered by at least an inch or two of water. The more eggs crowding the pan the more water you should have over the eggs. 6 eggs should be covered by at least an inch, 7 to 12 eggs, by 2 inches.

2. Heat the pot on high heat and bring the water to a full rolling boil. Adding a teaspoon of vinegar to the water may help keep the egg whites from running out if an egg does crack while cooking. Some people also find that adding 1/2 teaspoon of salt to the water helps prevent cracking as well as making the eggs easier to peel.

3. Turn off the heat, keep the pan on the hot burner, cover, and let it sit for 10 - 12 minutes. If you have the type of stove burner that doesn't retain heat when turned off, you might want to lower the temp to low, simmer for a minute, and then turn it off. Depending on how cooked you like your hard-boiled eggs, the eggs should be done perfectly in 10 - 12 minutes. That said, depending on your altitude, the shape of the pan, the size of the eggs, the ratio of water to eggs, it can take a few minutes more. Or, if you like your eggs not fully hard-cooked, it can take a few minutes less. When you find a time that works for you, given your preferences, the types of eggs you buy, your pots, stove, and cooking environment, stick with it. If you are cooking a large batch of eggs, after 10 minutes sacrifice one to check for doneness by removing it with a spoon, running it under cold water, and cutting it open. If it's not done enough for your taste, cook the other eggs a minute or two longer. Usually, it is very hard to overcook eggs by using this method. You can let the eggs sit, covered for up to 15 - 18 minutes without the eggs getting overcooked.

4. Strain the water from the pan and run cold water over the eggs to cool them quickly and stop them from cooking further. Or, if you are cooking a large batch of eggs, remove them with a slotted spoon to a large bowl of ice water. It's typically easier to peel the eggs under a bit of running water. The best way to store hard-boiled eggs is in a water-covered container in the refrigerator. Eggs can release odors in the fridge which is why it helps to keep them covered. They should be eaten within 5 days. The good thing about this method is that even if you forget them and the eggs sit in the water a few minutes longer than you had planned, they'll still be fine. Some people like their eggs less or more hard-cooked than others. If you want your eggs still a little translucent in the center, let them seep in the hot water for only 6 minutes or so.

Bone Broth
Prep Time: 25 minutes
Cook Time: 18+ hours
Total Time: 18+ hours & 25 minutes
Servings: 8

Ingredients
• 6 pounds beef bones
• ¼ cup apple cider vinegar (optional)

Instructions
1. Arrange the bones in a single layer in a large roasting tray and place them in the oven at 450°F (232°C) for about 20 minutes, until golden brown. Note: This step is optional and followed to affect the end flavor of the broth.
2. Place all bones in a large stockpot. Fill with enough water to fully cover the material.
3. Pour in the apple cider vinegar, if you decide to use it.
4. Bring the water to a boil, then reduce it down to a simmer. Adjust the flame and pot lid to maintain a low simmer.
5. Cook for at least 18 hours, and up to 72 hours. Most people pull their batch after about 24 hours. Check periodically to ensure the water remains over the bones. Add extra water as needed.
6. Let the broth cool slightly. If a layer of scum or film appears over the top, skim it off with a slotted spoon. Strain the broth through a fine-mesh strainer or cheesecloth. Store in glass jars in the fridge for up to 5 days or in the freezer for longer.

Pemmican
Prep Time: 20 mins
Total Time: 20 mins
Servings: 16 pieces

Ingredients
• 1 pound dried and ground meat

- 1 tablespoon salt
- 2 tablespoons herbs and spices (optional)
- 1 pound beef tallow melted

Instructions

1. Melt the tallow in an oven-safe container or double boiler over medium-low heat. At 350° F/175° C, it takes about 10 minutes in the oven.
2. Combine the meat, salt, and optional herbs and spices in a bowl.
3. Once the tallow is melted, but not too hot, pour over the dry material and combine well. There should be just enough tallow to moisten all the meat, but not make puddles. If the fat does not completely incorporate the dry meat, add a little more.
4. Mix well.
5. Transfer into an 8×8-inch baking dish to set.
6. Score into squares and store in an airtight container.

Notes

In place of cutting into squares, you may also roll the mixture in your hands like a meatball and form small balls. Silicon molds and standard or mini-muffin size pans are also useful for forming uniform-shaped pieces. Chocolate or soap molds can both be used for this purpose if they have a shape you like.

Pork Rinds (Chicharrones)

Prep Time: 30 minutes
Cook Time: 3 hours & 20 minutes
Total Time: 3 hours & 50 minutes

Ingredients
- 3 to 5 pounds pork back fat and skin
- Lard
- Sea salt to taste

Instructions

1. Preheat the oven to 250°F and set a wire rack over a baking sheet.

2. Using a very sharp knife, cut the pork skin and fat into long strips, about 2 inches wide. Score the fat on each strip every two inches. Insert knife carefully between skin and fat on one end of the strip and remove a portion of the fat (you will end up with a thin layer of fat still on the skin and that is fine).

3. Once that first part of fat is removed, you can hold the skin in one hand as you slide the knife down the strip to remove the majority of the fat. Again, a little fat still clinging to the skin is okay.

4. When the fat has been removed, cut each strip into 2-inch squares and place, fat-side down, on the wire rack.

5. Bake for 3 hours, until the skin is completely dried out.

6. Meanwhile, if you want to use the pork fat to cook your chicharrones, place it in a large saucepan over medium-low heat. Cook gently until most of the fat has liquified, about 2 hours. This is the same way you may also render pork fat for future cooking use. Use a slotted spoon to remove any remaining solids. Discard (or eat, they taste like bacon!).

7. When baking time is up, heat the lard to a depth of 1/3 in the pan. Or you may just have a few inches of lard and cook your pork rinds in batches. The cooking lard should be quite hot but not bubbling.

8. Add the pork rinds and cook until they bubble and puff up, about 3 to 5 minutes. Remove and drain on a paper towel-lined plate. Sprinkle immediately with salt.

Liver Chips

Prep Time: 5 minutes
Drying Time: 8 hours
Total Time: 8 hours & 5 minutes
Servings: 8 servings

Equipment (pick one)

• Food dehydrator
• Oven (optional)

Ingredients

• 1 pound beef liver ground or thinly sliced

Instructions

1. Use a spatula to spread the liver on a food dehydrator sheet or ovenproof baking sheet in one single layer. Stretch it out to make it as thin as possible.
2. Dry on the meat setting in the dehydrator. If you use an oven, set the heat at the lowest temperature possible.
3. Flip once the center is completely dry. This can take 8 - 12 hours in a food dehydrator, however, in the oven it will dry much more quickly, so check after an hour. Keep an eye on it until the edges separate and the center is dry.
4. Dry the second side thoroughly until no moisture remains.

Chicken Skin Cracklings

Prep Time: 10 minutes
Drying Time: 20 minutes
Total Time: 30 minutes
Servings: 4 servings

Ingredients

- 8 raw chicken skin pieces from thighs or breasts
- Salt and pepper
- Seasoning of your choice

Preparation

- Preheat oven to 400°F and place rack to middle position. Line a large rimmed baking sheet with parchment paper.

Instructions

1. Remove the chicken skin from the thighs or chicken breasts. Trim any large pieces of fat from the edges with a knife. Scrape away any extra fat or skin on the underside of the skin.
2. Dry the skins completely on paper towels and stretch out onto the parchment paper in a single layer.
3. Season lightly with salt and pepper or your favorite seasoning. Go easy because the chicken skin will shrink (as much as 50%) as it cooks, concentrating the seasoning. The chicken skin will fry in its own fat.
4. Bake for approximately 20 minutes or until browned and crisp. They should be a deep golden brown. Remove from the pan and drain excess fat on paper towels.

5. Cool completely and store in an airtight container in the fridge. Place on a sheet pan in a 350° F oven for several minutes to re-crisp if needed.

6. Makes 8 oven-fried chicken skin chips.

Bacon Cheese Chips

Tools
• Cookie sheet and spatula

Ingredients
• Shredded Cheese
• Nitrate-free bacon or hot dogs
• Beef Tallow

Instructions
1. Coat cookie sheet with beef tallow or lard.
2. Shred cheese.
3. Cook bacon until fully cooked and crispy.
4. Cut bacon into small pieces a.k.a. bacon bits.
5. Make small little circular piles of cheese on the cookie sheet and top with the bacon bits.
6. Pre-heat oven to 370° and when ready, place the cookie sheet in the oven and cook for around 8 minutes.
7. When fully cooked and crispy, let cool and cut out chips if necessary.

Cheese Crisps

Equipment
• Oven

Ingredients
• Your favorite semi-hard or hard cheese (i.e., Parmigiano, Grana Padano, Pecorino, Cheddar, Gruyere, Emmental, and Mimolette, etc)
• Seasoning (optional)

Instructions
1. Preheat oven to 350°F.
2. If using block cheese, cut the cheese into small uniform slices about ½ inch by 1 inch big.
3. Place pieces of cheese about 3 inches apart from each other onto a parchment-lined baking sheet.
4. If using shredded cheese pile about 2 teaspoons of shredded onto the parchment-lined baking sheet, keeping the piles about **3.** inches apart from each other. These will spread so do not put them close together or you will get one big mess.
5. If using seasoning, sprinkle the seasoning on top of the cheese.
6. Bake for about 15 - 20 minutes, until cheese has browned just a little bit. Times will vary with different cheeses and depending on how much is on the pan. Check them at 15 minutes.
7. Pull out of the oven and let cool for about 10 minutes before carefully removing from the pan.
8. Enjoy on top of meat or however you like.

Pepperoni Chips

Equipment
• Oven

Ingredients
• Organic pepperoni or thinly sliced dried meat/sausage

Instructions
1. Place pepperoni or meat/sausage slices on a parchment-lined sheet pan and bake for 18 - 20 minutes, flipping them halfway through.
2. Let cool. Chips will get crisp once cooled down.
3. Eat immediately. They do not stay crisp, but if you have leftovers you can re-crisp them in the oven for 3 - 5 minutes at 300 degrees.

Carnivore Muffins
Prep Time: 10 minutes
Cook Time: 20 minutes
Total Time: 30 minutes
Servings: 4 servings

Ingredients
• 9 large eggs
• 8 ounces ground beef
• 1 teaspoon salt

Instructions
1. Preheat the oven to 350°F (175°C).

2. Lightly grease a standard-size muffin tin.

3. Brown the meat in a skillet over medium heat.

4. Whisk eggs in a large bowl.

5. Add meat and salt. Stir to combine.

6. Remove from oven and cool for 5 minutes.

7. Release by running a knife around the edge of each muffin.

8. Pop out and continue cooling on a wire rack or serve.

9. Enjoy leftovers cold or reheat in the oven before serving.

Carnivore Charcuterie Board

Equipment
• Charcuterie Board

Ingredients
• 1 flat wooden cutting board or plank
• 2 - 4 different cheeses (about 2 - 3 ounces of each)
• 2 - 4 different cured meats (2 ounces of each)

Instructions
1. When selecting your cheeses try to get a combination of each one of the following styles: soft/mild cheese, hard sharp cheese, funky cheese, or specialty cheese.

2. When selecting your meats, choose your favorite deli meats or try something new. Charcuterie ideas: prosciutto, salami, mortadella, pastrami, bresaola, deli turkey and ham chunks.

3. When arranging your board, be sure all your components are different textures and cuts. For example, sliced prosciutto, diced ham chunks, sliced and rolled up mortadella, crumbled cheese, diced cheese, shaved cheese, etc.

4. Place each component on the board with some space in between each one. Do not cram everything right next to each other unless you only have a small platter.

5. If using a small board arrange meats and cheeses as close as possible starting from the inside of the plate to ensure the components are placed evenly throughout the board.

Simple Pâté

Servings: 4-8

Ingredients
• 12 - 16 oz liver (chicken liver is milder than beef liver)
• 8 oz bacon (beef or pork)
• 1/2 cup tallow (plus more if using fat to seal)
• 1 & 1/2 tsp salt
• 2 whole eggs, whisked

Instructions
1. Sauté bacon on medium heat in a cast-iron pan. Regular pan can work too.

2. After a few minutes of sauteing, add liver and cook until still pink inside.

3. Melt tallow.

4. Blend in everything, except eggs, in a blender or with a hand mixer.

5. As you are blending everything, pour in the eggs. Do not stop blending or else the eggs will scramble. Blend until smooth.

6. Store in jars. Seal the top of jars with extra melted fat to prevent oxidation.

7. Let chill to firm up and for the flavors to meld together.

9. Eat cold, spread some on a burger or cheese crisps. Or eat hot!

Beef Liver & Bacon Muffins

Equipment
• Oven

Ingredients
• 12 oz lean ground beef
• 12 oz beef liver
• 12 oz bacon (135 g cooked)
• ¼ cup bone broth
• 1 tsp oregano (optional)
• 1 tsp thyme (optional)
• 1 tsp rosemary (optional)
• 1 tbsp salt

Instructions
1. Preheat oven to 350°F.
2. Cook bacon, save bacon grease on the side for later use.
3. Blend cooked bacon and liver together.
4. Transfer to a large bowl and mix in the ground beef.
5. Add bone broth and spices.
6. Pour into a muffin pan & bake for roughly 30 minutes.

Bacon Weave

Ingredients
• 1 pack of nitrate-free bacon

Instructions
1. Preheat oven to 375°F.
2. Cut pack of bacon in half.
3. Using the half slices, lay 3 slices down in a row.
4. Lift the bottom of the middle slice halfway up and lay a piece of bacon down underneath it in the opposite direction. Lay the middle slice of bacon back down.
5. Lift the top of the 2 outer pieces halfway up and lay another piece of bacon down underneath them in the opposite direction. Lay the outer pieces back down.
6. Repeat with the rest of the bacon.
7. This should make 4 "slices" of bacon weave, but you may have to make a couple with only 4 pieces instead of 5, depending on how many slices are in your pack of bacon.
8. Bake on a sheet pan for 20 minutes.
9. Flip and cook for 5 more minutes.
10. Remove from oven and let cool before using.

Notes
You can also do this with the whole pack of bacon, without cutting it, so you can have a large bacon weave to wrap whatever your heart desires! You can wrap meatloaf, cheese stuffed chicken breast, or even a tenderloin.

Cornbread

Ingredients
- 10 ounces cooked chicken
- 6 whole eggs
- 2 ounces melted butter, plus extra for spreading on top
- ½ teaspoon baking soda
- ½ teaspoon salt

Instructions
1. Preheat oven to 350°F.
2. Blend all ingredients until smooth in a blender.
3. Grease your 4 cup casserole dish or bread pan with butter or line with parchment paper.
4. Depending on your pan, the bread will take about 40 minutes.
5. Check doneness at 30 minutes and if it is still wiggly and loose in the middle, let it continue cooking for 10 minutes.
6. Once you take the cornbread out of the oven, spread butter all over the top, as much as you want.

Carnivore Sandwich
Prep Time: 5 minutes
Cook Time: 5 minutes
Total Time: 10 minutes
Servings: 1 person

Ingredients
- 2 beef sausage patties
- 1 egg

- 1 oz cheddar cheese
- 1 teaspoon butter or bacon grease

Instructions

1. In a large skillet, melt butter over medium heat.

2. Form sausage into thin patties, about the size of your palm but only 1/2 inch thick.

3. Cook patties until they brown on one side, then flip, cooking for another 2 - 3 minutes, or until cooked through.

4. If you don't mind your food touching, fry an egg at the same time in the same pan. If not, you can use a little more butter in an additional pan (medium heat, and wait until the pan is hot to prevent sticking), and then assemble your carnivore breakfast sandwich. Keep the yolk runny, as your sauce.

5. To assemble, place one sausage patty on a plate, then top with fried egg, a slice of cheese, and another sausage patty.

Carnivore Black Pudding

Equipment

- Short cable tie wraps
- 2 funnels or 2 sausage making tubes (one larger than the other)
- An apron – just in case you spill or splash any of the blood!

Ingredients

- 500 g ground pork shoulder
- 50 g lamb liver – minced
- 50 g pig skin – minced
- 250 g pork back fat – diced

- 150 g dried pigs blood
- 600 ml water – warm
- 6 tsp sea salt
- Ox middles/bungs (these are large, edible and strong sausage casings)

Instructions

To prepare the pigskin:
1. Place in a large pan of boiling water and simmer for a couple of hours until soft.
2. Allow to cool and then place in a food processor to mince.
3. Set aside.

To prepare the liver:
1. Place in a food processor and mince.
2. Set aside.

To prepare the pork shoulder:
1. Either buy ground or cut into cubes and grind yourself with an electric grinder using the large grinding blade – make sure the meat is very cold as this will make it easier to grind.
2. Set aside.

To prepare the back fat:
1. Slice the fat into strips and then dice into small pieces.
2. Set aside.

To prepare the blood:

1. Measure 150g into a large jug and pour in 600ml of warm water and whisk until smooth.
2. Set aside.

To prepare the ox middles/bungs:
1. Soak in cold water for at least 20 minutes prior to use.

Making The Puddings:
1. Place all the pre-prepared meat ingredients into a large bowl and mix them together.
2. Slowly add the rehydrated blood, mixing it thoroughly (be careful not to splash it about or you will look like you are on a horror movie set!)
3. Add the salt and mix in.
4. Place another clean bowl next to your large bowl.
5. Roll the ox middles onto the funnel/largest sausage tube.
6. Use a cable tie wrap to close the end tightly.
7. Using a large serving spoon, start to carefully spoon the mixture into the funnel/tube and use the smaller sausage tube to push it down into the ox middle.
8. Use your other hand to guide the mixture into the ox middle, making sure there are no gaps or air pockets, feeding the pudding into the clean bowl.
9. Make sure that there is enough of liquid blood being added along with the meats.
10. Do not make each pudding too long before using another cable tie to close it off tightly, making sure that the pudding is firmly packed.
11. Leave a small gap in the ox middle (where you will later cut it) and then close off another section to start a new pudding.
12. Continue until all the mixture has been used.

---

13. Securely tie the last pudding and then cut each pudding between the cable ties to separate.
14. Bring a large pan of water to a boil.
15. Place the individual puddings into the water, turn down the heat and simmer for between an hour to an hour and a half.
16. Remove the puddings from the hot water and place immediately into a bowl of ice water and leave to cool.
17. Place into a dish and into the fridge overnight. Enjoy!

Scotch Eggs (Pork-Free)
Prep Time: 15 minutes
Cook Time: 25 minutes
Total Time: 40 minutes
Servings: 12 Scotch eggs

Ingredients
• 2 pounds ground beef or chicken sausage
• 2 teaspoons salt
• 12 large boiled eggs

Instructions
1. Preheat the oven to 350°F (175°C).
2. Line two small rimmed baking sheets with parchment paper.
3. Combine beef (or chicken) and salt in a large bowl. Use your hands to mix the ingredients together and form into 12 meatballs.
4. Place 6 meatballs on each of the lined baking sheets and press flat.
5. Place one boiled egg in the middle of each circle of meat and wrap the meat around the egg, leaving no gaps or holes.

6. Bake for about 15 minutes, turn them over, and continue for another 10 minutes, until outside is golden brown.

7. Place under the broiler to finish for 5 minutes for a crispy shell. Serve hot.

Homemade Raw Milk Yogurt

Prep Time: 10 minutes
Culture Time: 12 - 18 hours
Servings: 8 servings

Equipment
• 1 quart (liter) glass jar with lid
• Kitchen towel or cheesecloth
• Rubber band

Ingredients
• 4 cups raw milk
• 4 tablespoons raw milk yogurt mother culture

Instructions
1. Measure 4 cups of raw milk into a glass or plastic container.

2. Add 4 tablespoons of mother culture and mix well.

3. Cover with a towel or cheesecloth, secure with a rubber band.

4. Set on the counter in a warm spot about 70-77°F/20-25°C, out of direct sunlight.

5. Culture for 12-18 hours. Check by gently tilting the jar. If the yogurt separates from the side of the jar with a clean break, it is done. If it is still very liquid and pours up the side like milk, return it to the counter and check again later.

6. Once set, refrigerate for at least 6 hours before eating.

Notes
Follow the ratio of 1 tbsp of starter culture:1 cup raw milk, up to 8 cups per container.

Homemade Raw Butter

Ingredients
• Raw cream from raw milk*
• Sea salt

*You can buy raw cream directly or you can leave raw milk in the fridge for a few days until the cream separates at the top and then pull it.

Instructions
1. If you have raw milk, leave it in the fridge until the cream visibly separates to the top and then pull the cream.
2. Blend the cream for 5 or so minutes until more of a cottage cheese consistency.
3. Knead the butter under cold running water to separate it from the buttermilk.
4. Salt, store in the fridge & enjoy.

Main Dishes

Carnivore Meatballs With Beef Heart
Prep Time: 5 minutes

Cook Time: 20 minutes
Total Time: 25 minutes
Servings: 4

Equipment
• 8×8-inch square glass baking dish

Ingredients
• 8 ounces ground beef
• 8 ounces ground beef heart
• 1 teaspoon salt

Instructions
1. Mix the two ground meats in a bowl until well combined.
2. Season with salt.
3. Scoop approximately 2 ounces and roll between the palms of your hands to form a ball shape.
4. Place in a small glass baking dish.
5. Bake in a preheated oven at 350°F (175°C) for 20 minutes.
6. Juices will run onto the baking dish once the meat is cooked through.
7. Serve meatballs warm with this "sauce" spooned over.

Carnivore Steak Nuggets

Ingredients
• 1 pound venison steak or beef steak (cut into chunks)
• 1 large egg
• Lard

Carnivore Breading

- 1/2 cup grated parmesan cheese
- 1/2 cup pork rinds
- 1/2 teaspoon sea salt

Instructions

1. Combine the pork rinds, parmesan cheese and sea salt. Set aside.

2. Beat 1 egg. Place the beaten egg into a bowl and the breading mix in another.

3. Dip chunks of steak in egg, then in breading mix.

4. Place chunks on a wax paper-lined sheet pan or plate.

5. Freeze breaded raw steak bites for 30 minutes before frying. This helps to ensure that the breading will not lift when fried.

6. Heat lard to roughly 325 degrees °F.

7. Working in batches as necessary, fry steak nuggets (from frozen or chilled) until browned, about 2-3 minutes.

8. Transfer to a paper towel-lined plate, season with a sprinkle of salt, and serve.

Notes

You can make several batches of carnivore steak bites and store them raw in the freezer for up to 6 months.

Organ Meat Burger

Ingredients

- 16 oz ground beef
- 4 oz beef spleen
- 4 oz beef kidney

- 2 slices bacon (nitrate-free)
- 1 tbsp parsley (optional)
- 1 tsp oregano (optional)
- 1 tsp rosemary (optional)
- 3 tsp sea salt
- Beef tallow or butter

Instructions

1. Grind meat together, including bacon.

2. Mix in seasonings and salt.

3. Form into burgers.

4. Heat tallow or butter on a skillet.

5. Sear both sides of the burger to your liking. If you plan to freeze the burgers for later use, leave them pretty rare. This way, when you reheat the burgers, they will not be overcooked.

Beef Tongue (Crock Pot)

Equipment
- Crock Pot Slow Cooker

Ingredients
- 2 - 2.5 pounds beef tongue
- 1+ tsp sea salt
- Bay leaf (optional)

Instructions

1. Place beef tongue in crockpot & heavily season with salt. Add bay leaves if desired.

2. Pour in enough water to completely cover the beef tongue.

3. Set crockpot to low & cook for 8 hours, until the tongue is tender enough to poke through with a fork and come out easily.
4. Once finished, remove the beef tongue from the crockpot and allow it to cool.
5. Once cooked, place the beef tongue onto a working surface & begin to peel the outer layer of skin. It is much easier to peel the skin off after the tongue has been cooked, so you should be able to slit the skin with a knife and use your hands to peel.
6. Once cooled & peeled, using a fork, shred the beef tongue meat by scraping at the surface & 'pulling' down.
7. To keep the meat juicy, save the broth that was created in the crockpot & pour a desired amount over meat.

Organ Meat Pie

Prep Time: 15 minutes
Cook Time: 15 minutes
Total Time: 30 minutes
Servings: 4

Ingredients
• ½ pound ground beef
• ½ pound ground beef heart
• ½ pound ground beef liver
• Tallow or butter, ghee, or any other cooking fat
• 3 eggs
• Salt (to taste)

Instructions
1. Preheat oven to 350°F (175°C).

2. Lightly brown the meat in fat in a skillet over medium heat.

3. Combine all ingredients in a mixing bowl.

4. Salt to taste.

5. Pour evenly into a lightly greased 9-inch pie plate.

6. Bake for 15 minutes, until egg is set.

7. Remove from heat, cool for 5 minutes.

8. Serve warm and enjoy leftovers cold.

Parmesan-Pork Meatballs

Ingredients
- 2 pounds ground pork
- 1 cup shredded parmesan cheese
- 2 eggs (optional)
- 1 teaspoon sea salt

Instructions
1. Mix together the ground pork, parmesan cheese, and optional eggs. The cheese has plenty of salt, but you may want to cook a bit of the meat mixture in a pan on the stove and adjust the salt if needed - add 1 teaspoon of sea salt at a time until you get the saltiness that you like.

2. Preheat broiler to high. Raise the rack to the second slot down from the top in the oven. Line a metal baking tray with shallow sides (like a jelly roll pan) with parchment paper.

3. As the oven heats, roll meatballs into a desired size and place on the lined baking sheet; touching but not overlapping. Make sure your meatballs are all the same size so that they cook evenly.

4. Once preheated, broil the meatballs for 5 minutes, or until the tops start to darken. If you are freezing the meatballs, remove them now and cool, then transfer them to a freezer bag. Reheat/finish cooking from thawed, 350° for 20 minutes or until cooked through.

5. Move meatballs to the middle of the oven and turn the oven to 'bake' and 350° and bake for an additional 15 - 20 minutes, depending on how big your meatballs are.

6. To check doneness, cut a meatball in half. Slight pink in the middle is okay, as they will continue cooking as they cool.

7. Serve your meatballs, topping with more cheese as desired.

Tartare

Ingredients
- 12 ounces of lean beef (tenderloin, flank, sirloin, rump roast, etc.)
- 2 tsp brown or dijon mustard (optional)
- 1 tsp balsamic or apple cider vinegar (optional)
- 1 tsp salt
- 2 egg yolks

Instructions
1. If you want to dice the meat very, very tiny, then freeze meat for about 20 minutes.

2. Remove from freezer, slice into thin strips, then dice into tiny cubes.

3. In a bowl, combine all the ingredients and mix thoroughly.

4. Serve tartare in a bowl.

5. Serve by making a small dip in the top of the tartare mound and gently place the egg yolk on top.

6. Enjoy right away, leftovers do not hold well, as the meat gets mushy with the marinade.

Notes

Don't just limit yourself to beef. You may also try this recipe with other types of red meat, such as lamb, bison, or elk.

Crustless Mini Meat Pies (With Hidden Liver)

Prep Time: 10 minutes
Cook Time: 20 minutes
Total Time: 30 minutes
Servings: 12 mini pies

Equipment

• 12-cup muffin pan

Ingredients

• 1 pound ground beef
• ¼ pound ground beef liver
• 4 eggs
• 1 tablespoon tallow or other cooking fat
• 1 teaspoon salt
• 1 tablespoon herbs de Provence (optional)

Instructions

1. Preheat oven to 350°F / 175°C.
2. Combine meat and liver in a mixing bowl.
3. Add in eggs, stir well to combine.

4. Melt the tallow or cooking fat and add to meat.

5. Season with salt and optional herbs.

6. Grease a 12-cup muffin pan well or use cupcake liners.

7. Spoon mixture into each well evenly.

8. Bake for 20 minutes, until done.

9. Remove from oven and cool before removing.

10. Serve warm or enjoy leftovers cold.

Ground Beef Stroganoff

Prep Time: 5 minutes
Cook Time: 15 minutes
Total Time: 20 minutes
Servings: 8 servings

Ingredients
• Ground beef
• Beef bone broth
• Heavy whipping cream
• Salt

Instructions
1. Lightly brown the meat in a skillet over medium-high heat.

2. Break apart clumps with a spatula as needed.

3. Pour in bone broth and cream.

4. Season with salt.

5. Bring to a simmer and continue to cook for 5 - 10 minutes until liquid reduces by half.

6. Serve hot.

Cheesy Air Fryer Meatballs

Prep Time: 20 minutes
Rest Time: 12 minutes
Cook Time: 8 minutes
Total Time: 40 minutes
Servings: 4 meatball servings

Equipment
• Air Fryer

Ingredients
• 2 pounds ground beef
• 2 large eggs
• 2 ounces pork rinds
• 3 ounces shredded Italian cheese blend
• 1 tsp sea salt
• 1 tbsp lard or tallow

Instructions
1. Place all ingredients in a mixing bowl. With clean hands, knead the mixture until thoroughly combined.
2. Roll into balls approximately 1 ½ inches in diameter. This should make 24 meatballs.
3. Depending on the size of your air fryer, you'll cook them in batches.
4. Line your fryer basket with liners, if you use them. Otherwise, coat with cooking oil of your choice (i.e., butter, ghee, tallow, lard, etc).

5. Place meatballs in the basket, making sure they do not touch each other or the sides of the basket.

6. Cook at 350 degrees for 8 minutes. Pull out the basket and turn the meatballs over. Return to the air fryer and cook at 350 degrees for another 4 minutes.

7. Meatballs should reach an internal temperature of 165 degrees, and then they're done.

Braised Beef Shank

Prep Time: 5 minutes
Cook Time: 3 hours
Total Time: 3 hours & 5 mins
Servings: 4 servings

Ingredients

- 1 tablespoon beef tallow, butter, ghee, or any other cooking fat
- 4 pieces beef shank 1-inch thick, 8 ounces each
- 2 - 3 cups bone broth or water
- 1+ tsp salt

Instructions

1. Heat cooking fat in a cast iron or heavy bottom skillet with a lid or Dutch oven.

2. Brown both sides of the beef shanks, about 2 - 3 minutes per side, until a golden-brown crust forms.

3. Pour broth over shanks. Use at least 2 cups of broth. There should be enough broth to cover the meat ½ to ¾ of the way up the side.

4. Season with salt.

5. Bring it to a simmer. Reduce the heat and cover with a lid, but leave a small opening for the steam to escape.
6. Cook over low heat for 3 hours, until the meat falls off the bone. Serve warm in liquid.

Boiled Beef Kidney

Prep Time: 6 minutes
Cook Time: 8 minutes
Total Time: 14 minutes
Servings: 4 servings

Equipment
• Small pot with lid

Ingredients
• 1 beef kidney
• Salt (to taste)
• Butter

Instructions
1. Fill a small pot with enough water to submerge the kidney.
2. Cover and bring water to a boil over medium-high heat.
3. Reduce the heat, add kidney and leave the lid cracked to allow heat to escape.
4. Boil for 8 minutes, monitor the heat so water does not boil over.
5. Remove from heat, drain water and quickly rinse the kidney under cool water, if desired.
6. To serve, simply cut into half, medallions, or bite-sized pieces.

7. Sprinkle with optional salt to taste and eat with cold butter ad libitum.

Notes

Kidney fat is excellent and should be left on. Cooking time may vary due to the size of the kidney. Cooking time for the average beef kidney is 8 minutes. Extra-large ones may go for as long as 10 minutes. Lamb, sheep, and goat kidneys are smaller. They typically should be boiled for about 4 to 5 minutes. You want the kidney to boil for the full cooking time. Regulate temperature by adjusting the flame and setting the lid more or less cracked (open) to find the sweet spot of boiling, but not boiling over.

Carnivore Casserole with Ground Beef

Prep Time: 5 minutes
Cook Time: 25 minutes
Total Time: 30 mins
Servings: 4 servings

Ingredients

• 1 pound ground beef
• 6 large eggs
• ½ cup heavy cream
• 2 tablespoons cream cheese softened
• 1 teaspoon salt

Instructions

1. Preheat the oven to 350°F (175°C).
2. Lightly brown the meat in a skillet over medium heat.

3. Whisk the eggs in a large bowl.

4. Add the cream, cream cheese, and salt. Mix well to combine. Add meat and stir well.

5. Pour the egg-meat mixture into a greased 9-inch round pie plate or something similar.

6. Bake for 25-30 minutes until eggs set. Let rest for 10 minutes, then slice and serve.

Mozzarella-Stuffed Meatballs

Prep Time: 10 minutes
Cook Time: 25 minutes
Total Time: 35 minutes
Servings: 4 servings

Ingredients
• 2 pounds ground beef
• 1 tablespoon salt
• 8 ounces mozzarella cheese whole milk

Instructions
1. Preheat the oven to 350°F (175°C).

2. Mix the salt and meat in a bowl.

3. Cut the cheese into 8 cubes.

4. Divide the meat into 8 4-ounce balls. Make a well in the center of each ball and insert the cheese. Press the meat around to cover the hole and smooth over any lumps.

5. Arrange meatballs in a 9×13-inch glass baking dish or large cookie sheet with the seam up.

6. Bake for 25 minutes until cooked. Cool slightly and serve warm.

Carnivore Birthday Cake (Savory)

Prep Time: 15 minutes
Cook Time: 2 hours & 30 mins
Total Time: 2 hours & 45 mins
Servings: 12 servings

Ingredients

Braunschweiger (liver sausage):
• 1 ¼ pounds pork or beef liver
• ½ pound pork shoulder (or beef tongue)
• ¾ pound pork back fat
• 3 teaspoons sea salt
• 4 hard-boiled eggs

Decorations:

• 12 Slices of prosciutto or carpaccio
• 12 slices bacon (nitrate-free)

Instructions

1. Cut the pork/beef liver, pork shoulder and fat into cubes. Place into a food processor or blender and purée until you have a smooth purée.
2. Pack the purée into a 7-inch cake pan (spring-form works best) and cover tightly with foil making sure the foil lines the pan so the water doesn't get in. Place the pan in a roasting pan with an inch of boiling water and bake at 300 degrees °F for 2 hours or until meat is cooked but not browned; cook until the internal temperature of the meat reads 160 degrees °F.
3. Remove the loaf pan from the roasting pan. Use a spoon to 4 egg-sized holes into the meat. Place the hard-boiled eggs into

the meat and pat the meat back over the eggs. Let it completely cool in the cake pan. Refrigerate 1 to 2 days before using.

4. Remove the Braunschweiger from the cake pan. Prosciutto is often sticky enough to hold to the Braunschweiger. Use your hands to form the prosciutto around the meat cake.

5. Meanwhile make the bacon roses. To make the bacon roses you need 24 slices of bacon (2 slices per rose) and some toothpicks. Specifically, to make the bacon roses:

• Preheat oven or air fryer oven to 375 degrees °F.

• Place a piece of parchment on a rimmed baking sheet. Take one slice of bacon and roll it up like a jelly roll to make a cylinder shape. Take another slice of bacon to continue rolling around the rolled-up bacon to make a rose shape.

• Use a toothpick at the bottom of the rolled-up pieces of bacon rose to secure it. Place on the parchment-lined baking sheet so the cylinder is facing up.

• Repeat with remaining bacon.

• Place in the oven to bake for 30-40 minutes or until the bacon is cooked through and browned. If you use thin bacon, cook for 25-35 minutes; make sure to check often. If you use thick-cut bacon, cook for 35-45 minutes. Remove from oven and allow to cool a bit before handling.

6. Store in an airtight container in the fridge for up to 6 days.

Carnivore Pizza

Prep Time: 10 minutes
Cook Time: 25 - 30 minutes
Total Time: 35 - 40 minutes
Servings: 4 to 6 servings

Ingredients

For the crust:
- 1-pound ground chicken
- 1 beaten egg
- 1 cup shredded mozzarella
- 1/2 cup grated Parmesan
- 1/2 teaspoon salt
- 1 teaspoon Italian dried herbs (optional)
- 1/2 teaspoon garlic powder (optional)

For the carnivore pizza sauce:
- 2 tablespoons butter
- 1 cup heavy cream
- 1 cup grated parmesan cheese

For the toppings:
- 1 package uncured pepperoni
- 1 cup shredded mozzarella cheese

Instructions

To make the crust:

1. Preheat the oven to 450°F.

2. In a large bowl combine the chicken, egg, mozzarella, Parmesan, salt and optional herbs and garlic powder. Mix until well combined.

3. Line a baking sheet or pizza pan with parchment paper. Pour the crust mixture onto the pan and cover with a second sheet of parchment. This will keep your hands clean. Begin to press the mixture starting from the center moving outward, rotating the pan until the crust is pressed evenly in the shape desired and is 1/4-inch thick.

4. Place the crust in the preheated oven and bake for 15 - 18 minutes.

5. Remove the crust from the oven. There will likely be a little liquid in the pan. Use a few paper towels to soak this up.

6. Leave the oven on while you prepare the sauce.

To make the carnivore pizza sauce:

1. In a small saucepan, melt the butter over medium heat. Pour the cream into the melted butter and whisk bringing the butter and cream to a low boil. Whisk continuously for about 3 minutes allowing the cream to begin to thicken slightly.

2. Add the parmesan cheese to the hot cream and stir until the sauce is thickened and the cheese has melted. Remove from the heat. Set aside.

To assemble the pizza:

1. Pour the sauce on the pizza crust, covering evenly to the edges of the crust.

2. Arrange half of the pepperoni slices on the pizza. Sprinkle the shredded mozzarella on the pizza. Arrange the remaining pepperoni slices on top and place the pizza in the hot oven. Bake for an additional 7 to 10 minutes, or until the cheese has melted.

3. Remove from the oven, cut into slices, and serve immediately.

To refrigerate:

1. Store covered in the refrigerator for up to 3 days.

2. Reheat in a 350°F oven for 5 to 10 minutes, or in the microwave for 45 to 60 seconds.

Notes
You may use ground turkey in the place of chicken if you want.

Desserts

Carnivore Ice Cream

Ingredients
• 2 eggs
• 350 ml heavy whipping cream
• 1 tsp vanilla extract
• 2 tbsp raw honey

Instructions
1. First, separate the eggs yolks from the whites.
2. Whisk the egg yolks until smooth and fluffy and set them aside for later.
3. Combine the heavy whipping cream with vanilla extract and honey in a saucepan.
4. Bring to a boil and simmer until the cream thickens.
5. Set your burner to low heat and add the whipped egg yolks into the mixture.
6. Stir until the mixture thickens.
7. Let the mixture cool to room temperature then refrigerate.
8. Next, beat the egg whites until fluffy then fold into the cool cream mixture.

137

9. Pour the whole mix into a freezable tupperware or jar with a lid and place it in the freezer.

10. Stir occasionally and continue freezing until it reaches the desired consistency.

Raw Carnivore Ice Cream

Serving Size: 2 pints

Ingredients

- 2 cups raw cream
- 3 raw egg yolks
- 1/4 tsp sea salt
- 1 tbsp raw honey
- 1/4 tsp vanilla extract

Instructions

1. If you have raw milk, leave it in the fridge until the cream visibly separates to the top. Then pull the cream.

2. Blend the raw cream, yolks, and other additions.

3. Pour into a pre-frozen ice cream maker and allow to churn until thick.

4. Store in the fridge and enjoy.

Carnivore Cake (Sweet)

Prep Time: 10 minutes
Cook Time: 40 minutes
Total Time: 50 minutes
Servings: 9 servings

Ingredients
- 4 large eggs room temperature
- ½ cup raw honey
- 1 teaspoon vanilla extract
- 1¼ cups raw milk
- 5 tablespoons butter cubed

Instructions
1. Preheat the oven to 350°F (175°C).

2. Beat eggs on high in a large bowl for up to 5 minutes, until thickened.

3. Gradually add the honey, continue mixing until light and fluffy. Mix in vanilla.

4. In a small saucepan, heat milk and butter for about 2 minutes over medium heat, just until butter melts.

5. Slowly add to eggs, beat until combined.

6. Pour unit a greased 8×8-inch (20×20-cm) baking dish. Bake for 40 minutes until a toothpick inserted into the center comes out clean. Cool before serving.

Carnivore Waffles
Servings: 1 waffle

Ingredients
- 2 eggs
- 1/4 cup raw breakfast sausage (this cooks in the waffle iron just fine)
- Butter or lard
- Raw honey (optional)

Instructions

1. In a bowl crack the 2 eggs and whisk into the sausage. This will break the sausage into small bits so that it will cook evenly in the waffle iron.

2. Coat the waffle iron with some butter or lard.

3. Pour the contents into the hot waffle iron and close. Let cook for approximately 3 - 4 minutes.

4. Add some honey on top, if you choose to use it.

Carnivore Cheesecake (No Bake)

Prep Time: 10 minutes
Cook Time: 0 minutes
Total Time: 10 minutes
Servings: 1 serving

Ingredients

- 2 ounces cream cheese room temperature
- 1 tablespoon sour cream
- 1½ tablespoons heavy whipping cream
- ½ tablespoons raw honey
- ⅛ teaspoon vanilla extract

Instructions

1. Beat all ingredients together with an electric mixer. Continue mixing until smooth.

2. Serve immediately or chill for 30 - 60 minutes.

CHAPTER 6: CARNIVORE DIET FAQS

Why Does The Carnivore Diet Work So Well?

There is no doubt that this diet has helped thousands of people all over the world regain their health and vitality, lose weight, improve their body composition, athletic performance and start feeling great again. However, we need to sit back and rethink how an all-meat diet is able to promote healing to such a degree. Well, there are a few reasons behind the success of this primal diet approach:

• The carnivore diet contains minimal to no carbs, thus it helps restore the gut into balance. It alleviates dysbiosis and improves the composition of the gut microbiome.

• The carnivore diet is a very nutrient-dense diet filled with quality, healthy calories from fat and protein. It's particularly rich in minerals, fat-soluble vitamins (A, D, E, and K), and B complex vitamins.

• A strict, all-meat carnivore diet is the ultimate elimination diet, because it removes all foods that promote/exacerbate inflammation and chronic disease - processed sugar, synthetic food additives, refined carbohydrates, vegetable (seed) oils, anti-nutrients, and FODMAPs.

Who Should Follow The Carnivore Diet?

People belonging to the following groups should seriously consider following the carnivore diet:

• Those suffering from an autoimmune condition, or those looking to lower the levels of inflammation in their body.

• People wanting to lose weight or people wanting to improve their body composition.

Because the carnivore diet is an ultra low-carbohydrate diet, it gets rid of many of the problems that come with the standard American diet (SAD). Inflammation is reduced, autoimmunity diminishes, and excess weight goes away or is brought back to balance.

What Are The Potential Benefits Of The Carnivore Diet For Autoimmune Patients?

When done correctly, the potential benefits of the carnivore diet for all people, including autoimmune patients, include:

• Decreased systemic inflammation
• Increased energy levels
• Improved gut function
• Better concentration and cognitive performance
• Upregulated hormone production (cholesterol found exclusively in animal products is a precursor to all steroid hormones)
• Increased testosterone in men (diets rich in cholesterol and saturated fats increase androgen levels)
• Better weight management (weight gain or weight loss depending on the individual's needs)

• Better mental health (reduced stress, anxiety, and/or depression)

Can The Carnivore Diet Heal Autoimmune Disease?

Autoimmune disease is a lifelong battle. It can go into remission and lie there dormant, but it never completely goes away (e.g., you can always flare). However, achieving remission and keeping it that way will allow you to live a 100% symptom-free life, which is very similar to being a perfectly healthy, normal individual. The carnivore diet is a great, natural, non-invasive way to naturally manage and/or reverse autoimmune symptoms.

Additionally, it helps improve certain mental health conditions, such as chronic stress, anxiety and depression. In most cases, any diet that removes or minimizes toxins (both natural and synthetic), and increases vital nutrients will help someone manage whatever chronic health issues he/she is dealing with.

Is The Carnivore Diet Safe Long-Term?

The verdict on the safeness of the carnivore diet is not out yet. Historically, there have been (and still are) numerous cultures and tribes around the world that have thrived on meat-based diets. These people were and are in perfect health with zero signs of cancer, cardiovascular disease, diabetes, and other chronic, degenerative diseases.

What has been repeatedly shown though, is that once these tribes start to incorporate more Western foods into their diet, their microbiomes start to gradually shift and their health begins to deteriorate.

The primary reason that most people and health professionals consider the carnivore diet to be unhealthy is because animal foods are by default higher in saturated fats and cholesterol than plant foods. Basing their beliefs on correlation (and not causation) studies, these people accuse saturated fats and cholesterol of being responsible for various chronic degenerative diseases, including cardiovascular disease, diabetes, and cancer, while ironically, most studies point to processed sugar and seed (vegetable) oils being responsible for the majority of chronic diseases that plague the modern man, including cardiovascular disease, diabetes and cancer.

What Are The People's Results From Using The Carnivore Diet?

The results so far are quite impressive. To get a first-hand idea yourself, spend some time online reviewing other people's testimonials and experiences of following the carnivore diet for some time. In that way, you will get real feedback on this dietary approach and how it has helped tens of thousands of patients all over the world regain their health and vitality. There are many videos on Youtube where people talk about their 'carnivore diet experience' and how it has helped them overcome serious, lifelong, chronic, 'incurable' health problems, such as depression, anxiety, type II diabetes, obesity, and various autoimmune conditions.

What's The Easiest Way to Start The Carnivore Diet?

The easiest way to get started with the carnivore diet is to dedicate 1 to 4 weeks. If you are very ready to commit to this new lifestyle, try it for a full month. If you are nervous and inexperienced with dieting in general, try it for a week and decide from there. When you first start, keep it as simple as possible - do some grass-fed ground beef (1 cup) 2 - 3 times per day with some tallow or grass-fed butter, if you choose to include dairy. Butter. especially from goat or sheep, is one of the most nutritious, anti-inflammatory, autoimmune-friendly types of dairy products you can consume. Do this for 5 days and see how you feel. You will probably feel pretty good and notice that inflammation from whatever chronic/autoimmune issue you are dealing with has greatly diminished.

In most cases, the key to minimizing autoimmune symptoms is to keep your diet as simple, clean, nutritious and gut-friendly as possible. That translates to a diet low in pro-inflammatory foods and high in anti-inflammatory, nutrient-dense foods, such as meat. Ideally, you should follow such a diet until your symptoms completely dissipate. Then, all you have to do is to sustain healing for as long as possible.

Is Meat Healthy?

Meat is a superfood that has been a staple in the human diet for millions of years. The reason most people consider eating a lot of meat unhealthy is because, at the end of the day, we've been taught since we were little children by both our mother and doctor that meat (especially red meat) is bad for us and that we need fiber and vegetables to stay healthy.

Unfortunately, oftentimes, even experienced health professionals make ridiculous claims that are completely erroneous and set their patients for serious problems down the road. Countless people have suffered permanent and horrible side effects and complications after trusting and listening to the advice of their trusted doctor or personal physician. Of course, what we say here isn't that you shouldn't follow the advice of your primary care doctor or personal physician; but just to take everything you listen or hear with a grain of salt. Always filter information, apply critical thinking and investigate yourself, especially when it comes to sensitive issues, such as your health and well-being.

If the experts' claims about meat being the "bad guy" were actually true, then why are we suffering unprecedented levels of chronic/autoimmune disease, despite minimizing its consumption? New diseases and conditions pop up literally every day. Despite that, treatment options and solutions remain limited to drugs and surgery.

Most people intuitively know that meat is not bad for them. Actually, the first major evolutionary change in the human diet was the incorporation of meat and marrow from large animals, which occurred by at least 2.6 million years ago. Essentially, we've been eating meat for millions of years. We enjoy its taste, how it makes us feel, and how it satiates our hunger. We also enjoy how eating meat doesn't mess with our blood sugar levels and doesn't throw us into a "food coma" (like carbs do), even when eating large amounts of it.

Do We Really Need Vegetables To Stay Healthy?

Humans have thrived on a variety of diets with some of them including large amounts of vegetables to virtually no vegetables. Therefore, the answer to this question is very subjective and varies from individual to individual.

In most cases, people suffering from multiple autoimmune conditions have a) compromised digestion b) unhealthy gut microbiomes, and thus do not tolerate very well raw vegetables, especially early on in their healing journey. As their gut function and microbial diversity gradually return back to balance, these people can tolerate more and more vegetables (always well-cooked).

Every autoimmune patient needs to be very mindful of his/her symptoms and how he/she feels with and without vegetables, and adjust the diet accordingly.

What About Fiber On The Carnivore Diet?

When most people decide to embark on their first 1-month carnivore diet trial, they get really worried about bowel movements and not getting enough fiber. Then, they get really surprised when a few days later their bowel movements are perfectly normal. Actually, it's not uncommon after the first week or so on the carnivore diet to even see "perfect trophy poops" based on the Bristol stool chart.

Good-consistency bowel movements may continue for the rest of the month, which makes a lot of people wonder about the importance of fiber. Most of us believe that we need fiber to increase our stool volume and scrub our intestines while coming out.

However, eating fiber is not always in our best interest. For example, there are studies showcasing that reducing your dietary fiber intake can help alleviate or reduce symptoms of chronic constipation. Obviously, the types of fiber and their source do play a role in these situations, however, eating more fiber is not always the solution when dealing with constipation (as most people are advised by their doctors).

Fiber exerts its beneficial effects in ways that most people fail to acknowledge. For example, supports digestive health by acting as a prebiotic for our beneficial intestinal bacteria. Our gut bacteria love to feast on prebiotic fibers, which help them multiply and produce beneficial metabolites, such as short-chain fatty acids (SCFAs), also found in butter.

Fiber also helps improve the quality and integrity of our mucus gut barrier. This is a thick mucus layer in our gut that separates intestinal bacteria from our actual gut wall. If the bacteria have no fiber to eat, they may start eating and digesting that mucus layer, ending up stimulating our immune system. That's why it is fair to say that fiber has its benefits and drawbacks. A good general piece of advice when it comes to including or not including fiber in your diet is to stay very mindful of how your body reacts to it. Not all people have the same reaction or tolerance to fiber, and we shouldn't condemn anyone who decides to include it in his/her diet.

Is The Carnivore Diet Ketogenic?

Most of the time, yes. When following a strict, all-meat carnivore diet you will be in a state of nutritional ketosis for the majority of time. Now you may say "a high protein intake can kick you out of ketosis due to glyconeogenesis taking place in the liver," which is correct but isn't always the case when following carnivore. Many carnivores have tested themselves out on multiple occasions while eating a meat-only diet and surprise, surprise, they were still in ketosis, despite their excessively high protein intake.

Most usually, it's the absence of carbohydrates that drives ketosis. Some people even choose to use a protein-sparing modified fast (PSMF) and still remain in ketosis. PSMF is a great strategy for dropping body fat, while retaining some muscle mass. In most cases, an all-meat carnivore diet is stricter and lower in carbs than your standard ketogenic diet where 30 - 50 grams of net carbs are allowed per day.

Can The Carnivore Diet Cause Nutrient Deficiencies? If Yes, How To Prevent Them?

While a muscle meat-only carnivore diet can be problematic from a nutrition standpoint, most of the nutrients lacking can be found in organ meats - liver, kidney, sweetbreads, lungs, brain, and so on. Thus, the key to preventing nutrient deficiencies when following an all-meat carnivore diet is to include enough organ meats (offal). Some of the best options include:

Liver

Liver is the "king" of organ meats. It is a powerful dietary source of bioactive vitamin A (retinol) and nutrients such as folate (vitamin B9), vitamin B12, and zinc. Vitamin A is particularly beneficial for eye health and for reducing your risk of various chronic, inflammatory diseases, including everything from Alzheimer's disease to arthritis. Liver also contains heme iron, chromium, copper, and zinc, and is known to be particularly beneficial for the heart, and increasing hemoglobin levels in the blood.

Kidney

Rich in nutrients and high-quality protein, kidney meat contains omega-3 fatty acids and the enzyme diamine oxidase (DAO). DAO is a histamine-degrading enzyme that helps get rid of allergic symptoms. Lack of DAO may cause problems, such as histamine intolerance and constant allergies. Eating kidney is additionally known to offer systemic anti-inflammatory benefits and to be good for the heart.

Brain

Brain contains omega-3 fatty acids (especially DHA) and other nutrients beneficial for our brain. Among these nutrients are phosphatidylcholine and phosphatidylserine, which are very important for the health of our nervous system. On top of that, the antioxidants obtained by eating brain meat are particularly effective in protecting the human brain and spinal cord from free radical damage.

Heart

Heart is rich in folate (vitamin B9), iron, zinc, and selenium. It is also a great source of vitamins B2, B6, and B12, all three of which belong to a group known as B complex vitamins. B vitamins found in organ meats exert cardioprotective effects, meaning they help prevent heart disease. B vitamins are also associated with maintaining healthy blood pressure, reducing high cholesterol, and forming new, healthy blood vessels. B vitamins are beneficial for the brain and have been found to reduce the risk of Alzheimer's disease, dementia, depression, and anxiety. Additionally, heart meat is a great source of coenzyme Q10 (CoQ10). This coenzyme functions as an antioxidant and has been shown to help treat and prevent certain diseases, particularly heart conditions. CoQ10 has also been shown to slow down the aging process and improve energy levels.

Tongue

Tongue meat is rich in calories and fatty acids, as well as iron, zinc, choline, and vitamin B12. This meat is considered particularly beneficial for those recovering from illness or pregnant women. Folate (vitamin B9) is the vitamin in organ meats considered to be particularly beneficial for fertility and for helping to prevent fetal defects in babies, such as spina bifida and heart problems. In addition, vitamin B6 (pyridoxine) present in tongue meat has been shown to be particularly helpful during the morning sickness phase of pregnancy.

Does The Carnivore Diet Increase Serum Cholesterol?

It can, but not always. Your liver creates and clears cholesterol from your blood. Your diet accounts for a relatively small percentage of the cholesterol found in your bloodstream. Some individuals (about 33% of the population) notice their serum cholesterol raising after increasing their dietary cholesterol intake. These people are known as hyper-responders and should manage how much cholesterol they take in through diet. For the rest 67% of the population though, there is no correlation between dietary cholesterol and hypercholesterolemia (abnormally high cholesterol in the blood), which is why the current US dietary guidelines no longer limit consumption of dietary cholesterol to 300 mg per day.

Can The Carnivore Diet Cause Constipation?

Yes, the carnivore diet can cause constipation, but diarrhea is actually the more common digestive problem most people deal with. It's worth noting here that what many individuals consider to be "carnivore constipation" is in actuality just fewer bowel movements. This is because the carnivore diet is a low-residue diet that contains no fiber. Most of the meat is digested higher up in the digestive tract with fewer waste products being left over for elimination. On top of that, since there is no dietary fiber to absorb water, body fluids have to exit in some way and the colon is a common route of elimination.

What Are The Most Common Digestive Problems When First Starting The Carnivore Diet?

There is no definite answer to this question. The most common digestive problem most people deal with when first starting is diarrhea because their body is trying to adapt to processing more dietary fat. The lack of fiber and carbs that naturally absorb water exacerbate that issue.

Diarrhea may also occur due to salt overconsumption (i.e., oversalting your meals or water). If you suspect that you suffer from fat malabsorption, then supplements like ox bile or pancreatic lipase can prove very beneficial for helping you break down and absorb dietary fats. If you have fat malabsorption issues, know that raw fat (uncooked) digests better than cooked or rendered fat, and is more anti-inflammatory.

Can Eating Too Much Meat Cause Kidney Problems?

The scientific consensus on the protein-kidney health connection is that high-protein diets can indeed be problematic for people already suffering from chronic kidney disease (not healthy people), and that low-to-moderate protein diets are generally advisable for CKD patients.

However, just because a low-protein diet can be beneficial for those with already-existing kidney issues doesn't mean a high-protein diet causes kidney disease in the first place. Generally, it's the processed meats that are very high in additives and preservatives like nitrates and sodium derivatives (i.e., monosodium glutamate - MSG) that are nephrotoxic. Additionally, in some cases, excessive amounts of dietary salt, especially if processed, may also overburden the kidneys as these organs struggle to flush the excess sodium out.

That's why processed meats in general, despite their palatability and convenience, are not ideal for chronic disease recovery.

It's also important, no matter what diet you follow, to ensure an adequate intake of water, so your body can dilute metabolic byproducts and toxins, and remove them through urination. An adequate intake of water helps the kidneys to maintain homeostasis and get rid of accumulated wastes.

How Long Does It Take To Adapt To The Carnivore Diet?

It usually takes about 10 - 30 days to adapt to the diet and enter full ketosis. Depending on your previous dietary habits, how strict you choose to be, and your levels of physical activity, this can take as long as 2 weeks.

Can I Use Supplements When Following The Carnivore Diet?

Yes, some supplements may be included while on the carnivore diet. Ideally, you should avoid any products containing carbohydrates. Supplements, such as a multivitamin or desiccated liver capsules are a good option, at

CARNIVORE DIET FOR BEGINNERS

least in the initial stages, until you get more knowledgeable and educated on the nutritional profile of various animal foods.

Does The Carnivore Diet Work For Athletes?

The carnivore diet can work for athletes, especially those suffering from chronic gut or autoimmune issues. If you are someone with a long history of high starch consumption (i.e., bread, pasta, rice, potatoes, etc) you should expect a small dip in energy, strength, stamina, and athletic performance for the first few weeks, simply due to the depletion of glycogen. However, once your body fully adapts and enters ketosis, you'll be able to get all the energy, strength and stamina you need from a new and superior source of fuel - fat and ketones.

Can You Build Muscle While On The Carnivore Diet?

Yes, you can build muscle while following the carnivore diet. Actually, more and more people are coming to the conclusion that a carnivore style of eating is one of the best ways to achieve lean muscle growth (building muscle while gaining minimal fat). With the perfect mix of fat, protein, cholesterol, creatine, vitamins and minerals, you'll have everything you need to gain the most optimal results from your training.

Is Weight Loss Easier On The Carnivore Diet?

In most cases, yes. As with all diets though, you'll need to pay some attention to your overall energy balance (calories in vs calories out). Most people who follow the carnivore diet achieve their weight loss goals very easily by simply eating liberal amounts of meat, oftentimes much more than they expected.

Is it a Good Idea to Eat Meat as a Pre-Workout Meal?

There are a few things you need to consider about eating meat as a pre-workout meal. Unlike the usual carb-rich meal you eat before you workout, meat takes a lot more time to be fully digested by your body. That's because meat is a nutrient-dense, chemically-complex food that requires a decent amount of time to be fully broken down by your digestive system. So, to get the maximum benefits of eating meat as a pre-workout meal, try to eat it at least an hour to an hour and a half before your training.

Can You Eat Carbs While On The Carnivore Diet?

This is a popular question. Ideally, no. You shouldn't eat any carbs while on the carnivore diet - with very few exceptions. In most cases, carbohydrates will mess up with your blood sugar and ketone levels.

One of the primary goals of following the carnivore diet is to eliminate carbohydrates altogether and get your metabolism into fat-burning and healing mode as much as possible. If you are an athlete or someone who wants to put on some weight, or someone that simply chooses to follow a more carnivore-ish (not 100% strict carnivore) approach, you may include some animal foods higher in carbs, such as raw dairy and honey.

What Is The Best Diet For Healing Autoimmunity?

There isn't one "best" diet for putting an autoimmune condition into remission. There are many dietary strategies you can use to manage and/or reverse autoimmune symptoms. In all cases and no matter the diet you choose to follow, you need to be very mindful of how your body reacts to particular foods, as well as what type of foods make you feel and function the best.

Do not become self-righteous or allow yourself to be bossed around by other people who think that their way works the best. There simply isn't one perfect universal diet or formula that works well for everyone. There are some common denominators among diets that work very efficiently for reducing inflammation and promoting systemic health. These diets usually:

• Include healthy sources of fat
• Have a low sugar content
• Remove gluten and wheat
• Minimize or remove lectins
• Remove processed dairy products, especially cow dairy
• Normalize gut dysbiosis by restricting starchy carbohydrates

Some of the most successful dietary approaches for healing chronic/autoimmune disease include:
• Carnivore Diet
• Keto Diet
• Paleo Diet
• AIP Diet*
• GAPS diet
• Primal Diet
• SCD (Specific Carbohydrate Diet) Diet
Regardless of which approach you choose to follow, you can tweak it according to your own individuality and genetics, and achieve great results!

*Check out *The Simple AIP (Autoimmune Protocol) Handbook: An Ancestral Approach to Fix Leaky Gut and Reverse Autoimmunity Through Nourishing Foods* by George Kelly for more.

CONCLUSION

The carnivore diet is a simple, yet powerful dietary approach for losing weight and managing/reversing chronic disease. It's a diet based almost entirely on animal products, particularly meat, such as beef, lamb, bison, poultry, and pork. Eggs and dairy products are also sometimes allowed depending on the carnivore diet variation and strictness. Fatty cuts of meat, such as ribeye, New York strip, Delmonico, etc, and organ meats (offal), such as liver, heart and tongue, are particularly desirable in this diet because they are extremely nutrient-dense.

The primary goal of the carnivore diet is to restore health and vitality to the body by addressing nutrient deficiencies and eliminating inflammatory foods that may irritate the gut and stimulate the immune system. Some people call the carnivore diet a 'zero-carb' diet, because it includes virtually no carbohydrates. This is especially true when the diet is comprised only of meat. The carnivore diet is considered by many a more extreme version of the ketogenic diet, which also includes very few carbohydrates and emphasizes nutrient density.

Anecdotally, the carnivore diet has been shown to be particularly effective for healing gut permeability or "leaky gut syndrome," which is considered by many alternative and functional medicine doctors a primary instigator in the manifestation of autoimmune disease. The mainstream medical world is quite resistant to accepting "leaky gut syndrome" as a primary causative factor in autoimmunity. Despite that, autoimmune patients all over the world try the carnivore diet and see the results for themselves. There are so many amazing stories out there that it's simply hard to deny the benefits of the diet.

By eating 100% strict carnivore, you eliminate the majority of dietary toxins and antigens - both synthetic and natural - that could otherwise irritate your gut and stimulate your immune system in a negative way. You also supply your body with vitally important nutrients, such as amino acids, essential fatty acids, cholesterol, minerals, trace elements, enzymes, and other co-factors not found in plant foods that are crucial for restoring proper gut function, intestinal barrier integrity, and overall health.

Future scientific studies, reports, and interventions will hopefully shed light on why and how the carnivore diet is so effective at managing, reversing, and even healing 'incurable' chronic diseases.

Your Opinion Matters

Did this book help you in some way?
If so, we'd love to hear about it!
Scan the QR code below to leave your honest review.

Scan here!

REFERENCES

Chapter 1

1. Megan R. Ruth et al., *"Consuming a hypocaloric high fat low carbohydrate diet for 12 weeks lowers C-reactive protein, and raises serum adiponectin and high density lipoprotein-cholesterol in obese subjects,"* Metabolism. 2013 Dec; 62(12): 10.1016/j.metabol.2013.07.006.
2. Tara Kelly et al., *"Low-Carbohydrate Diets in the Management of Obesity and Type 2 Diabetes: A Review from Clinicians Using the Approach in Practice,"* Int J Environ Res Public Health. 2020 Apr; 17(7): 2557. Published online 2020 Apr 8.
3. Lisa Quigley et al., *"The complex microbiota of raw milk,"* FEMS Microbiology Reviews, Volume 37, Issue 5, September 2013, Pages 664–698.
4. Dominik H Pesta et al., *"A high-protein diet for reducing body fat: mechanisms and possible caveats,"* Nutr Metab (Lond). 2014; 11: 53. Published online 2014 Nov 19.
5. Jaecheol Moon et al., *"Clinical Evidence and Mechanisms of High-Protein Diet-Induced Weight Loss,"* J Obes Metab Syndr. 2020 Sep 30; 29(3): 166–173. Published online 2020 Jul 23.
6. Mona Mohamed Ibrahim Abdalla, *"Ghrelin – Physiological Functions and Regulation,"* Eur Endocrinol. 2015 Aug; 11(2): 90–95. Published online 2015 Aug 19.

7. David Furman et al., *"Chronic inflammation in the etiology of disease across the life span,"* Nat Med. 2019 Dec; 25(12): 1822–1832. Published online 2019 Dec 5.
8. Roma Pahwa et al., *"Chronic Inflammation,"* StatPearls [Internet].
9. Robert Oh et al., *"Low Carbohydrate Diet,"* StatPearls [Internet].
10. Insaf Berrazaga et al., *"The Role of the Anabolic Properties of Plant- versus Animal-Based Protein Sources in Supporting Muscle Mass Maintenance: A Critical Review,"* Nutrients. 2019 Aug; 11(8): 1825. Published online 2019 Aug 7.
11. Andrew J. Murray et al., *"Novel ketone diet enhances physical and cognitive performance,"* FASEB J. 2016 Dec; 30(12): 4021–4032. Published online 2016 Aug 15.
12. Kristin L. Osterberg et al., *"Carbohydrate exerts a mild influence on fluid retention following exercise-induced dehydration,"* J Appl Physiol (1985) . 2010 Feb;108(2):245-50.

Chapter 2

1. Wajeed Masood et al., *"Ketogenic Diet,"* StatPearls [Internet].
2. Susan A. Masino et al., *"Mechanisms of Ketogenic Diet Action,"* National Center for Biotechnology Information (US); 2012.
3. Giovanna Muscogiuri et al., *"The management of very low-calorie ketogenic diet in obesity outpatient clinic: a practical guide,"* J Transl Med. 2019; 17: 356. Published online 2019 Oct 29.
4. Victoria M. Gershuni et al., *"Nutritional Ketosis for Weight Management and Reversal of Metabolic Syndrome,"* Curr Nutr Rep. 2018 Sep; 7(3): 97–106.

5. Adriano Bruci et al., *"Very Low-Calorie Ketogenic Diet: A Safe and Effective Tool for Weight Loss in Patients with Obesity and Mild Kidney Failure,"* Nutrients. 2020 Feb; 12(2): 333. Published online 2020 Jan 27.

Chapter 3

1. Winston J Craig, *"Health effects of vegan diets,"* Am J Clin Nutr . 2009 May;89(5):1627S-1633S.
2. Olga Yeliosof et al., *"Veganism as a cause of iodine deficient hypothyroidism,"* J Pediatr Endocrinol Metab . 2018 Jan 26;31(1):91-94.
3. Vesanto Melina et al., *"Position of the Academy of Nutrition and Dietetics: Vegetarian Diets,"* J Acad Nutr Diet . 2016 Dec;116(12):1970-1980.
4. Alex Ankar et al., *"Vitamin B12 Deficiency,"* Treasure Island (FL): StatPearls Publishing; 2021 Jan.
5. Lisa A. Riesberg et al., *"Beyond Muscles: The Untapped Potential of Creatine,"* Int Immunopharmacol. 2016 Aug; 37: 31–42. Published online 2016 Jan 8.
6. Mojtaba Kaviani et al., *"Benefits of Creatine Supplementation for Vegetarians Compared to Omnivorous Athletes: A Systematic Review,"* Int J Environ Res Public Health. 2020 May; 17(9): 3041. Published online 2020 Apr 27.
7. Guilherme Giannini Artioli et al., *"Carnosine in health and disease,"* Eur J Sport Sci . 2019 Feb;19(1):30-39.
8. Rathish Nair et al., *"Vitamin D: The "sunshine" vitamin,"* J Pharmacol Pharmacother." 2012 Apr-Jun; 3(2): 118–126.
9. Omeed Sizar et al., *"Vitamin D Deficiency,"* Treasure Island (FL): StatPearls Publishing; 2021 Jan.

10. J Christopher Gallagher et al., *"Dose response to vitamin D supplementation in postmenopausal women: a randomized trial,"* Ann Intern Med . 2012 Mar 20;156(6):425-37.

11. Johann Diederich Ringe et al., *"Vitamin D-insufficiency,"* Dermatoendocrinol. 2012 Jan 1; 4(1): 72–80.

12. Caroline Richard, *"Docosahexaenoic Acid,"* Adv Nutr. 2016 Nov; 7(6): 1139–1141. Published online 2016 Nov 10.

13. Fady Moustarah et al., *"Dietary Iron,"* Treasure Island (FL): StatPearls Publishing; 2021 Jan.

14. Nazanin Abbaspour et al, *"Review on iron and its importance for human health,"* J Res Med Sci. 2014 Feb; 19(2): 164–174.

15. Stephen Schaffer et al., *"Effects and Mechanisms of Taurine as a Therapeutic Agent,"* Biomol Ther (Seoul). 2018 May; 26(3): 225–241. Published online 2018 Apr 10.

16. David Rogerson, *"Vegan diets: practical advice for athletes and exercisers,"* J Int Soc Sports Nutr. 2017; 14: 36. Published online 2017 Sep 13.

17. Yoichiro Ishida, *"Vitamin K2,"* Yoichiro Ishida.

18. David Rabinovich et al., *"Zinc,"* Treasure Island (FL): StatPearls Publishing; 2021 Jan.

19. Meika Foster et al., *"Effect of vegetarian diets on zinc status: a systematic review and meta-analysis of studies in humans,"* J Sci Food Agric. 2013 Aug 15;93(10):2362-71.

Chapter 4

1. Reetta Satokari, *"High Intake of Sugar and the Balance between Pro- and Anti-Inflammatory Gut Bacteria,"* Nutrients. 2020 May; 12(5): 1348. Published online 2020 May 8.

2. Yuanqing Gao et al., *"Dietary sugars, not lipids, drive hypothalamic inflammation,"* Mol Metab. 2017 Aug; 6(8): 897–908. Published online 2017 Jun 20.
3. Alena Fajstova et al., *"Diet Rich in Simple Sugars Promotes Pro-Inflammatory Response via Gut Microbiota Alteration and TLR4 Signaling,"* Cells. 2020 Dec; 9(12): 2701. Published online 2020 Dec 16.
4. Bhaskar Bhardwaj et al., *"Death by Carbs: Added Sugars and Refined Carbohydrates Cause Diabetes and Cardiovascular Disease in Asian Indians,"* Mo Med. 2016 Sep-Oct; 113(5): 395–400.
5. Vincent R Franceschi et al., *"Calcium oxalate in plants: formation and function,"* Annu Rev Plant Biol . 2005;56:41-71.
6. S C Noonan et al., *"Oxalate content of foods and its effect on humans,"* Asia Pac J Clin Nutr . 1999 Mar;8(1):64-74.
7. Weiwen Chai et al., *"Effect of different cooking methods on vegetable oxalate content,"* J Agric Food Chem . 2005 Apr 20;53(8):3027-30.
8. Aristo Vojdani, *"Lectins, agglutinins, and their roles in autoimmune reactivities,"* Altern Ther Health Med . 2015;21 Suppl 1:46-51.
9. Lan Shi et al., *"Changes in levels of phytic acid, lectins and oxalates during soaking and cooking of Canadian pulses,"* Food Res Int . 2018 May;107:660-668.
10. Saieda M. Kalarikkal et al., *"Breastfeeding,"* Treasure Island (FL): StatPearls Publishing; 2021 Jan.
11. Artemis Dona et al., *"Health risks of genetically modified foods,"* Crit Rev Food Sci Nutr. 2009 Feb;49(2):164-75.

Chapter 6

1. David O. Kennedy, *"B Vitamins and the Brain: Mechanisms, Dose and Efficacy—A Review,"* Nutrients. 2016 Feb; 8(2): 68. Published online 2016 Jan 28.
2. Adarsh Kumar et al., *"Role of coenzyme Q10 (CoQ10) in cardiac disease, hypertension and Meniere-like syndrome,"* Pharmacol Ther . 2009 Dec;124(3):259-68.
3. Mario Festin et al., *"Nausea and vomiting in early pregnancy,"* BMJ Clin Evid. 2009; 2009: 1405. Published online 2009 Jun 3.
4. F L Santos et al, *"Systematic review and meta-analysis of clinical trials of the effects of low carbohydrate diets on cardiovascular risk factors,"* Obes Rev . 2012 Nov;13(11):1048-66.
5. Luc Djoussé et al., *"Dietary cholesterol and coronary artery disease: a systematic review,"* Curr Atheroscler Rep . 2009 Nov;11(6):418-22.
6. Ronald P Mensink et al., *"Effects of dietary fatty acids and carbohydrates on the ratio of serum total to HDL cholesterol and on serum lipids and apolipoproteins: a meta-analysis of 60 controlled trials,"* Am J Clin Nutr. 2003 May;77(5):1146-55.
7. Allon N. Friedman et al., *"Independent influence of dietary protein on markers of kidney function and disease in obesity,"* Kidney International Volume 78, Issue 7, 1 October 2010, Pages 693-697.
8. Helga Frank et al., *"Effect of short-term high-protein compared with normal-protein diets on renal hemodynamics and associated variables in healthy young men,"* Am J Clin Nutr. 2009 Dec;90(6):1509-16.
9. Stephen P. Juraschek et al., *"Effect of a High-Protein Diet on Kidney Function in Healthy Adults: Results From the*

OmniHeart Trial," Am J Kidney Dis. 2013 April; 61(4): 547–554.

10. William F Martin et al., *"Dietary protein intake and renal function,"* Nutr Metab (Lond). 2005; 2: 25.

11. Allon N Friedman et al., *"Comparative effects of low-carbohydrate high-protein versus low-fat diets on the kidney,"* Clin J Am Soc Nephrol. 2012 Jul;7(7):1103-11.

12. Hercules Sakkas et al., *"Nutritional Status and the Influence of the Vegan Diet on the Gut Microbiota and Human Health,"* Medicina (Kaunas). 2020 Feb; 56(2): 88. Published online 2020 Feb 22.

13. Neil J Mann, *"A brief history of meat in the human diet and current health implications,"* Meat Sci . 2018 Oct;144:169-179.

About The Author

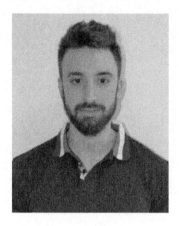

George Kelly

George Kelly is a registered dietitian nutritionist (RDN) that specializes in chronic, autoimmune conditions. His mission is to help people all over the world regain their health, wellness, vitality and confidence. You can join his AIP diet support group at www.facebook.com/groups/aiphealing

Printed in Great Britain
by Amazon

33554734R00096